DISABILITY STUDIES

INTELLECTUAL DISABILITY

SOME INTERNATIONAL ASPECTS

DISABILITY STUDIES

Joav Merrick - Series Editor –

NATIONAL INSTITUTE OF CHILD HEALTH
AND HUMAN DEVELOPMENT,
MINISTRY OF SOCIAL AFFAIRS, JERUSALEM

Intellectual Disability: Some International Aspects
Ariel Tenenbaum and Joav Merrick (Editors)
2020. ISBN. 978-1-53617-866-1 (Softcover)
2020. ISBN. 978-1-53617-867-8 (e-book)

Pain Management Yearbook 2017
Joav Merrick (Editors)
2018. ISBN: 978-1-53613-693-7 (Hardcover)
2018. ISBN: 978-1-53613-694-4 (e-book)

Quality of Life and Intellectual Disability: Knowledge Application to other Social and Educational Challenges
Roy I. Brown and Rhonda M. Faragher (Editors)
2014. ISBN: 978-1-62948-264-4 (Hardcover)
2018. ISBN: 978-1-53613-063-8 (Softcover)
2014. ISBN: 978-1-62948-272-9 (e-book)

Parkinson's Disease: Awareness among Young Adults
Ronald Chow, Jaclyn Viehweger, Michael Borean, Drew Hollenberg, and Joav Merrick (Editors)
2017. ISBN: 978-1-53612-745-4 (Hardcover)
2018. ISBN: 978-1-53612-745-4 (Softcover)
2017. ISBN: 978-1-53612-746-1 (e-book)

Human Development: Equipping Minds with Cognitive Development
Carol T. Brown and Joav Merrick
2018. ISBN: 978-1-53613-053-9 (Softcover)
2018. ISBN: 978-1-53613-054-6 (e-book)

Autism Spectrum Disorder: Awareness among Young Adults
Ronald Chow, Jaclyn Viehweger, Joav Merrick (Editors)
2017. ISBN: 978-1-53612-730-0 (Hardcover)
2017. ISBN: 978-1-53612-731-7 (e-book)

Virtual Reality: Recent Advances in Virtual Rehabilitation System Design
Wendy Powell, Albert "Skip" Rizzo, Paul M. Sharkey and Joav Merrick
2017. ISBN: 978-1-53612-040-0 (Softcover)
2017. ISBN: 978-1-53612-061-5 (e-book)

Child Abuse: Children with Disabilities
Vincent J Palusci, Dena Nazer, Donald E Greydanus and Joav Merrick
2017. ISBN: 978-1-53612-035-6 (Hardcover)
2017. ISBN: 978-1-53612-056-1 (e-book)

Rehabilitation: Innovations and Challenges in the Use of Virtual Reality Technologies
Wendy Powell, Albert "Skip" Rizzo, Paul M. Sharkey and Joav Merrick, (Editors)
2017. ISBN: 978-1-53612-080-6 (Hardcover)
2017. ISBN: 978-1-53612-099-8 (e-book)

Virtual Reality: Recent Advances for Health and Wellbeing
Wendy Powell, Paul M Sharkey and Albert "Skip" Rizzo
2017. ISBN: 978-1-53612-454-5 (Softcover)
2017. ISBN: 978-1-53612-455-2 (e-book)

Pediatric Pain: Current Aspects
Hatim A. Omar, Dilip R. Patel, Donald E. Greydanus, and Joav Merrick (Editors)
2016. ISBN: 978-1-63485-505-1 (Hardcover)
2016. ISBN: 978-1-63485-537-2 (e-book)

Recent Advances on Using Virtual Reality Technologies for Rehabilitation
Paul M. Sharkey and Joav Merrick (Editors)
2016. ISBN: 978-1-63484-027-9 (Hardcover)
2015. ISBN: 978-1-63484-028-6 (e-book)

Technology, Rehabilitation and Empowerment of People with Special Needs
Lena Pareto, Paul M Sharkey and Joav Merrick (Editors)
2015. ISBN: 978-1-63482-713-3 (Hardcover)
2015. ISBN: 978-1-63482-737-9 (e-book)

Virtual Reality: Rehabilitation in Motor, Cognitive and Sensorial Disorders
Paul M. Sharkey and Joav Merrick (Editors)
2014. ISBN: 978-1-63321-773-7 (Hardcover)
2014. ISBN: 978-1-63321-787-4 (e-book)

Virtual Reality: People with Special Needs
Paul M. Sharkey and Joav Merrick (Editors)
2014. ISBN: 978-1-63321-729-4 (Hardcover)
2014. ISBN: 978-1-63321-734-8 (e-book)

Intellectual Disability: Some Current Issues
Joav Merrick, Donald E Greydanus and Dilip R. Patel (Editors)
2014. ISBN: 978-1-63321-855-0 (Hardcover)
2014. ISBN: 978-1-63321-867-3 (e-book)

From One Century to the Next: A History of Wrentham State School and the Institutional Model in Massachusetts
Ingrid Grenon
2014. ISBN: 978-1-63117-711-8 (Hardcover)
2014. ISBN: 978-1-63483-805-4 (Softcover)
2014. ISBN: 978-1-63117-712-5 (e-book)

Pain and the Elderly
Joav Merrick and Mimi M.Y. Tse
2013. ISBN: 978-1-62948-468-6 (Hardcover)
2013. ISBN: 978-1-62948-475-4 (e-book)

Pain: International Research in Pain Management
Joav Merrick, Patricia Schofield and Mohammed Morad (Editors)
2013. ISBN: 978-1-62948-423-5 (Hardcover)
2013. ISBN: 978-1-62948-435-8 (e-book)

Disability and Chronic Disease
Joav Merrick, Shoshana Aspler and Mohammed Morad (Editors)
2013. ISBN: 978-1-62948-288-0 (Hardcover)
2013. ISBN: 978-1-62948-307-8 (e-book)

Down Syndrome and Dementia. A Comprehensive and Historical Review
Vee P. Prasher
2012. ISBN: 978-1-62081-263-1 (Hardcover)
2012. ISBN: 978-1-62081-271-6 (e-book)

Rett Syndrome: Therapeutic Interventions
Meir Lotan and Joav Merrick (Editors)
2011. ISBN: 978-1-61728-614-8 (Hardcover)
2011. ISBN: 978-1-61728-080-1 (Softcover)
2011. ISBN: 978-1-61761-131-5 (e-book)

Pain Management Yearbook 2010
Joav Merrick (Editor)
2011. ISBN: 978-1-61209-972-9 (Hardcover)
2011. ISBN: 978-1-62808-255-5 (e-book)

Pain Management Yearbook 2009
Joav Merrick (Editor)
2011. ISBN: 978-1-61209-666-7 (Hardcover)
2011. ISBN: 978-1-62081-774-2 (e-book)

Pain. Brain Stimulation in the Treatment of Pain
Helena Knotkova, Ricardo Cruciani and Joav Merrick (Editors)
2011. ISBN: 978-1-60876-690-1 (Hardcover)
2011. ISBN: 978-1-61470-495-9 (e-book)

Neural Plasticity in Chronic Pain
Helena Knotkova, Ricardo A. Cruciani and Joav Merrick (Editors)
2011. ISBN: 978-1-61324-657-3 (Hardcover)
2011. ISBN: 978-1-62417-407-0 (e-book)

Disability from a Humanistic Perspective: Towards a Better Quality of Life
Shunit Reiter
2011. ISBN: 978-1-60456-412-9 (Hardcover)
2011. ISBN: 978-1-63117-654-8 (e-book)

Cancer in Children and Adults with Intellectual Disabilities: Current Research Aspects
Daniel Satgé and Joav Merrick (Editors)
2011. ISBN: 978-1-61761-856-7 (Hardcover)
2011. ISBN: 978-1-61122-187-9 (e-book)

Contemporary Issues in Intellectual Disabilities
V. P. Prasher
2010. ISBN: 978-1-61668-023-7 (Hardcover)
2010. ISBN: 978-1-61209-292-8 (e-book)

DISABILITY STUDIES

INTELLECTUAL DISABILITY

SOME INTERNATIONAL ASPECTS

ARIEL TENENBAUM, MD

AND

JOAV MERRICK, MD, MMEDSCI, DMSC

EDITORS

nova
Medicine & Health
New York

Library of Congress Cataloging-in-Publication Data

Names: Tenenbaum, Ariel, editor. | Merrick, Joav, 1950- editor.
Title: Intellectual disability: some international aspects / [edited by] Ariel Tenenbaum, Joav Merrick.
Description: New York: Nova Science Publishers, [2020] | Series: Disability studies | Includes bibliographical references and index. | Summary: "Developmental disabilities or neurodevelopmental disabilities (includes intellectual disability) are a diverse group of chronic disorders that begin at anytime during the development process (including conception, birth, and growth) up to 22 years of age and last throughout an individual's lifetime. Major disabilities include intellectual disabilities, learning disabilities, communication disorders, autism spectrum disorders, cerebral palsy, and neural tube defects. We provide an introduction and review epidemiology of major disabilities and have also gathered international research from United States, Australia, Ghana, Jordan, Ireland, Italy and India on various aspects of intellectual and developmental disability, which we hope will be of interest to our readers"-- Provided by publisher.
Identifiers: LCCN 2020016518 (print) | LCCN 2020016519 (ebook) | ISBN 9781536178661 (paperback) | ISBN 9781536178678 (adobe pdf)
Subjects: LCSH: Intellectual disability--Cross-cultural studies.
Classification: LCC RC570 .I464 2020 (print) | LCC RC570 (ebook) | DDC 362.3--dc23
LC record available at https://lccn.loc.gov/2020016518
LC ebook record available at https://lccn.loc.gov/2020016519

Published by Nova Science Publishers, Inc. † New York

CONTENTS

INTRODUCTION

In: Intellectual Disability
Editors: Ariel Tenenbaum et al.
ISBN: 978-1-53617-866-1

Chapter 1

INTELLECTUAL, DEVELOPMENTAL AND NEURODEVELOPMENTAL DISABILITIES

Dilip R Patel[1,*], MD, Ariel Tenenbaum[2-4], MD and Joav Merrick[3-6], MD, MMedSci, DMSc

[1]Department of Pediatrics and Human Development, Michigan State University College of Human Medicine, Kalamazoo Center for Medical Studies, Kalamazoo, Michigan, United States of America
[2]Center for Children with Chronic Diseases and Down Syndrome Center Jerusalem, Israel
[3]Department of Pediatrics, Mt Scopus Campus, Hadassah Hebrew University Medical Center, Jerusalem, Israel
[4]National Institute of Child Health and Human Development, Jerusalem, Israel

* Corresponding Author: Professor Dilip R Patel, MD, MD, FAAP, FACSM, FSAM, FAACPDM, Chair, Department of Pediatrics and Human Development, Michigan State University College of Human Medicine, Kalamazoo Center for Medical Studies, Kalamazoo, Michigan, MSU/ KCMS/ Pediatrics, 1000, Oakland Drive, Kalamazoo, MI, United States. E-mail: patel@kcms.msu.edu.

[5]Kentucky Children's Hospital, University of Kentucky, Lexington, Kentucky, United States of America
[6]Center for Healthy Development, School of Public Health, Georgia State University, Atlanta, Georgia, United States of America

Abstract

Developmental disabilities or neurodevelopmental disabilities (includes intellectual disability) are a diverse group of chronic disorders that begin at any time during the development process (including conception, birth, and growth) up to 22 years of age and last throughout an individual's lifetime. Major disabilities include intellectual disability, learning disabilities, communication disorders, autism spectrum disorders, cerebral palsy, and neural tube defects. This chapter provides an introduction and reviews epidemiology of major disabilities. In this book we have gathered international research from researchers in the United States, Australia, Ghana, Jordan, Ireland, Italy and India on various aspects of intellectual and developmental disability, which we hope will be of interest to our readers.

Introduction

Developmental disabilities or neurodevelopmental disabilities (includes intellectual disability) are a diverse group of chronic disorders (see Table 1) that begin at any time during the development process (including conception, birth, and growth) up to 22 years of age and last throughout an individual's lifetime (1). The underlying basis for these disorders lies in fundamental deficits in the developing brain due to genetic, prenatal, perinatal, metabolic, and other factors (2). Developmental disabilities affect 17% of individuals younger than 18 years of age in the United States (1). Prevention along with early recognition and intervention are critically important to mitigate the enormous personal and socioeconomic impact of these disorders.

Table 1. Major categories of developmental disabilities

Intellectual disability
Learning disabilities
Communication disorders
Autism spectrum disorders
Neurobehavioral disorders
Neurogenetic disorders
Neurometabolic disorders
Neuromuscular disorders
Cerebral palsy
Other neuromotor disorders
Sensory impairments
Disabilities associated with chronic diseases
Traumatic brain injuries
Spinal cord injuries

The World Health Organization has developed the International Classification of Functioning, Disability, and Health (ICF), which consists of three key components – body function and structure, activity, and participation – that provides a framework for delineating disabilities (see Table 2) (2, 3). The three key components of functioning and disability are inter-related and may interact with the health condition (e.g., disorder or disease) and personal and environmental factors.

Table 2. World Health Organization international classification of functioning, disability and health

Normal function	Lack of normal function
Body function: The physiological functions of the body	Impairment: Problems in the body function as a significant deviation or loss
Body structures: Anatomic parts of the body	Impairments: Problems in structure as a significant deviation or loss
Activity: The execution of a task or action by an individual	Activity limitation: Difficulties an individual may have in executing activities
Participation: Involvement in a life situation	Participation restrictions: Problems an individual may have in involvement in life situation
Functioning: A global term used to encompass body functions, body structures, activities, and participation	Disability: A global term used to encompass problems with body functions, body structures, activity limitations, and participation restrictions

http://www.who.int/classifications/icf/en/.

In the United States, according to the Individuals with Disability Education Improvement Act (2004) the term child with a disability means a child with intellectual disability, hearing impairments (including deafness), speech or language impairments, visual impairments (including blindness), serious emotional disturbance, orthopedic impairments, autism, traumatic brain injury, other health impairments, or specific learning disabilities (4). A child with disability as defined by the IDEA needs special education and related services, as may be required to assist a child with a disability to benefit from special education, and includes the early identification and assessment of disabling conditions in children.

The term infant or toddler with a disability means an individual under three years of age who needs early intervention services because she or he is experiencing developmental delays, as measured by appropriate diagnostic instruments and procedures in one or more of the areas of cognitive development, physical development, communication development, social or emotional development, and adaptive development; or has a diagnosed physical or mental condition that has a high probability of resulting in developmental delay.

According to the Americans with Disabilities Act (ADA) the term 'disability' means, with respect to an individual – a physical or mental impairment that substantially limits one or more major life activities of such individual; a record of such an impairment; or being regarded as having such an impairment (5). Major life activities include, but are not limited to, caring for oneself, performing manual tasks, seeing, hearing, eating, sleeping, walking, standing, lifting, bending, speaking, breathing, learning, reading, concentrating, thinking, communicating, and working. A major life activity also includes the operation of a major bodily function, including but not limited to, functions of the immune system, normal cell growth, digestive, bowel, bladder, neurological, brain, respiratory, circulatory, endocrine, and reproductive functions.

INTELLECTUAL DISABILITY

According to the American Association of Intellectual and Developmental Disabilities (AAIDD), intellectual disability "is a disability characterized by significant limitations both in intellectual functioning and in adaptive behavior as expressed in conceptual, social, and practical adaptive skills" (6, 7). The assessment of intellectual functioning and adaptive behavior must take into consideration the expectations based on individual's age and culture (8). The influence on cognitive assessment of sensory, motor, communication, or behavioral factors should also be appropriately considered in administration of assessment instruments, and interpretation of their results (8).

In the United States a widely used definition is the one from the IDEA that defines intellectual disability as "significantly sub-average general intellectual functioning, existing concurrently with deficits in adaptive behavior and manifested during the developmental period that adversely affects a child's educational performance"(4). According to the Diagnostic and Statistical Manual of Mental Disorders, 4th edition, text revision (DSM-IV-TR), intellectual disability (or mental retardation) is defined as an intelligence quotient (IQ) of approximately 70 or below on an individually administered standardized test of intelligence concurrent with deficits in adaptive functioning in two of the following areas: communication, self-care, home living, social or interpersonal skills, use of community resources, self-direction, functional academic skills, work, leisure, health, and safety. All definitions stipulate that the onset of disability must occur before the age of 18 years (9-11).

The severity of intellectual disability can be categorized based on a combination of level of intellectual functioning, adaptive functioning, and intensity of supports needed (8, 9, 12). When the level of intellectual functioning cannot be reliably assessed, but there is a high level of confidence based on clinical judgment, a diagnosis of intellectual disability can be made without specifying the severity of intellectual functioning (7, 8).

The reported prevalence of intellectual disability reflects consideration of the definition used, method of ascertainment of the data, and the characteristics of the population studied (13, 14). Based on the typical bell shaped distribution of intelligence in the general population and two standard deviations below the mean as a cut off point, approximately 2.5% of the population is expected to have intellectual disability. Most epidemiological studies consider those with an IQ score of 50 or less as having severe and those above 50 as having mild intellectual disability (10-15). Eighty five percent of individuals with intellectual disability have mild intellectual disability (9-12). The prevalence of severe intellectual disability has remained the same over several decades at 0.3%-0.5% of the population in the United States (12). Based on the United States National Center for Health Statistics 1997-2003 National Health Interview Survey, the prevalence of intellectual disability among children ages 5-17 years is estimated to be 7.5 per 1,000 (12). Intellectual disability is reported to be twice as common in males as in females. The recurrence risk of intellectual disability in families with one previous child with severe intellectual disability is reported to be between 3% and 9% (8, 11, 12).

Mild intellectual disability is associated predominantly with environmental risk factors and a specific etiology can be identified in less than half of affected individuals (12-14). On the other hand, underlying biological or neurological etiology can be identified in more than two-thirds of affected individuals who have severe disability (8, 11, 13). The most common identified conditions in children with severe intellectual disability include chromosomal disorders, genetic syndromes, congenital brain malformations, neurodegenerative diseases, congenital infections, inborn errors of metabolism, and birth injury (12-14).

Learning disabilities

The term learning disability describes difficulties in specific areas of learning that have a direct relation to academic performance. The terms learning disabilities (LDs) and learning disorders are often used interchangeably in the literature. The main types of learning disabilities are reading disability (dyslexia), mathematics disability (dyscalculia), disorder of written expression (dysgraphia), and non-verbal learning disability (NVLD) (16, 17). The failure to achieve academically in children who have LDs occurs in the presence of age-appropriate teaching and learning experiences, and is not the result of cognitive deficits or sociocultural factors (16, 17). Early identification is crucial to prevent academic failure, behavioral disturbances, low self-esteem, early school dropout, and lifelong implications for academic success, occupation, socioeconomic well being and consequently health.

A child is considered to have a specific learning disability if the child does not achieve adequately for the child's age or to meet grade-level educational standards in one or more of the specific areas, when provided with learning experiences and instruction appropriate for the child's age or State approved grade level standards (4).

To ensure that underachievement in a child suspected of having a specific learning disability is not due to the lack of appropriate instruction in reading or math, the following must be taken into consideration, as part of the evaluation: data that demonstrate that prior to, or as a part of, the referral process, the child was provided appropriate instruction in regular education settings, delivered by qualified personnel; and data-based documentation of repeated assessments of achievement at reasonable intervals, reflecting formal assessment of student progress during instruction, which was provided to the child's parents (4). The public agency must promptly request parental consent to evaluate the child to determine if the child needs special education and related services.

Specific LD is diagnosed when the child or adolescent's scores on an individually administered standardized achievement test (in reading, mathematics, or written expression) are substantially below that expected based on his or her age, level of education, and IQ. Because LDs can occur at all levels of IQ the definitional concept of discrepancy between ability and achievement is an area of controversy and debate in the LD literature (4, 16, 17).

Specific reading disability is fairly common, with up to 17.5% of children being affected (18, 19). Dyslexia is highly comorbid with other developmental problems, including impairments in language, motor skills, and behavioral control (20). Reading disability is also a contributor to juvenile delinquency, and leads to higher rates of recidivism (21). Dyslexia is identified in 80% of children who have LDs.

Specific mathematics disorder (also known as dyscalculia) is also fairly common, seen in 3%-6% of school-age children (22-24). It is more common in girls than in boys, possibly related to environmental, rather than biological, factors. The presence of dyscalculia should prompt physicians to look for medical and psychiatric syndromes, given that mathematics disorder is present at higher-than-average rates in conditions such as epilepsy and fragile X syndrome (22-26).

Of the all LDs, the disorder of written language (also called written-language disorder, or WLD) is the least researched (27, 28). However, a study from Minnesota found that, by age 19 years, 6.9%-14.7% of the subjects met criteria for WLD, which is about as common as reading disorder (27). Boys with WLD outnumbered girls 2-3:1 and 25% of all subjects had WLD without a comorbid reading disorder.

Communication disorders

Language is a system of symbolic knowledge represented in the brain used for meaningful communication. The English language has 44 phonemes. A phoneme is a unit of sound in speech. A Morpheme (word) refers to the smallest meaningful unit of language. Speech is the production of sounds of words. Communication disorders are common in school-age children identified in 12-14% of students. In school age children the prevalence of expressive language disorder is reported to be 3-7%, and mixed receptive-expressive disorder to be 3-5%. (9). The reported prevalence of phonologic disorder I 2% by 6-7 y of age and 0.5% by 17 y of age and that for stuttering ranges 0.8-1.0% in adolescents (9).

AUTISM SPECTRUM DISORDERS

Autism spectrum disorders (ASDs) are a group of developmental disabilities characterized by significant deficits in social, communication, and behavioral domains (29, 30). Autistic disorder, Asperger syndrome, and pervasive developmental disorder not otherwise specified (PDD NOS), are the 3 ASDs. Persons who have autistic disorder have significant language delays, social and communication challenges, and unusual behaviors and interests (30). A significant percentage of them also have intellectual disability. Persons who have Asperger syndrome manifest deficits in social domain and have unusual behaviors and interest; however, they typically do not have deficits in language or intellectual ability. Persons with pervasive developmental disorder – not otherwise specified, have some features of autistic disorder and some features of Asperger syndrome, but do not meet all the criteria for either disorder (30).

Centers for Disease Control and Prevention reports that the overall prevalence of ASDs in the United States is 9.0 per 1 000 population in children aged eight years (29). The average prevalence of ASDs is four times higher in males than in females (30). The risk for a second child having an ASD, when an older sibling has ASD, is 5%-6% (29, 30). In the United States, the average prevalence of ASDs identified among children aged 8 years has increased by 57% from 2002 to 2006.42 The prevalence of ASDs has increased 10 fold over the past 50 years (29, 30). Although various reasons have been postulated for the increased prevalence, the exact reasons have not been clearly elucidated (3-32).

Of the estimated four million children born in the United States each year approximately 27,000 will eventually be diagnosed with ASD (30). Assuming a constant prevalence rate over the past 20 years, approximately 600 000 persons between the ages of 0 and 21 have an ASD (30-33). The prevalence rate of ASD in Asia and Europe is reported to be between 0.6% and 1% (30-33).

There is high covariance between the ASDs and IDs, as between 50% and 70% of individuals with ASDs will have some type of ID; conversely, as many as 40% of those with IDs will have an ASD (34). In children with

IDs, the most reliable prevalence rate of comorbid pervasive developmental disorders (PDDs) is 16.7%, which was derived using DSM-IV-TR criteria (9, 35). The ASD-ID combination tends to increase the severity of both disorders, leading to more subjective distress, less functional ability, and greater need for community services.

No cause is found in most cases of ASDs (36, 37). There are some genetic syndromes, both common (e.g., Down syndrome and fragile X syndrome) and rare (e.g., adenylosuccinate lyase deficiency), that are associated with higher-than-expected rates of autism (51). It is unclear if there is something inherent in those syndromes that predisposes to the development of autistic features, or whether the risk is secondary to the intellectual impairment that is commonly seen in many genetic disorders.

Cerebral palsy

According to American Academy of Cerebral Palsy and Developmental Medicine cerebral palsy (CP) describes a group of permanent disorders of development of movement and posture, causing activity limitation, that are attributed to nonprogressive disturbances that occurred in the developing fetal or infant brain (39, 40). The motor disorders of CP are often accompanied by disturbances of sensation, perception, cognition, communication, and behavior, by epilepsy, and by secondary musculoskeletal problems. CP is classified as spastic (hemiplegia, diplegia, quadriplegia), dyskinetic (choreoathetoid, dystonia), hypotonic, or mixed (39-41).

The worldwide incidence of CP is estimated to be 2 to 3 per 1,000 live births (39, 42-44). Each year about 10,000 babies born in the US develop CP (45). Because initial symptoms and signs suggestive of CP may resolve during first few years of life, the prevalence of CP is generally higher in infancy. Despite a tremendous improvement in obstetric and neonatal care, the overall prevalence of CP has remained the same since the 1950s (40, 41). This trend is partly explained by the fact that most low birth weight and premature babies now survive. Although, prematurity and low birth weight are significant risk factors for developing CP, multiple other risk factors have been identified (39-46).

MYELOMENINGOCELE

Neural tube defects (NTDs) result from failure of the neurulation that is failure of the closure of the neural tube during development of central nervous system as expected between the 3rd and 4th week of in utero development (47, 48). Although, any segment of spinal level can be affected, 75% of cases involve the lumbosacral level (49). Myelomeningocele is the most severe type of NTD in which there is a defect in the vertebral column through which the meninges and the spinal cord protrude at the level of the defect (48).

The prevalence of NTDs varies in different regions of the world (49). In the United States, the incidence of NTDs is 1 in 4 000 live births (47, 49). In Wales and Ireland, the prevalence is 3 to 4 times higher, whereas in Africa it is much lower (49). The variability in prevalence rates of NTDs in different regions of the world is believed to be due to a combination of genetic and environmental factors. Lumbar myelomeningocele, which is 3-7 times more common in females than in males, accounts for most cases of myelomeningocele (47-49).

A significant decrease (50%) in the prevalence of NTDs has been reported over the past 4 decades (49). Some of the reasons believed to have contributed to the decrease in prevalence of NTDs include routine and widespread supplementation with folic acid, prenatal diagnosis and subsequent decision to terminate pregnancy by some couples, and improved nutrition as well as general health of women (47, 49).

Dual diagnosis

The reported prevalence rates of psychiatric disorders in persons who have developmental disabilities have been quite inconsistent, depending on the studies' choice of variables, such as subject age (child, adolescent, adult or elderly), setting (clinical or community), location (family home, residential care or state hospital), degree of intellectual impairment (mild, moderate or severe), developmental diagnosis (specific developmental syndrome vs. non-specific etiology), psychiatric diagnosis (specific disorders vs. grouped as "mental illness"), and evaluation method (chart review, survey or clinical interview). Another important challenge to the accurate measurement of psychopathology in the developmental disabilities is the difficulty in differentiating psychiatric symptoms from the clinical features associated with some of the developmental disabilities themselves (50-55). Taking these technical issues into consideration, the rates of some behavioral and emotional disorders do appear to be higher in the persons who have developmental disabilities than they are in comparison groups ranging from 20%-50% (51-55).

Hearing loss

Sounds can be described in terms of their frequency (or pitch) and intensity (or loudness). Frequency is measured in hertz (Hz). A person, who has hearing within the normal range, can hear sounds that have frequencies between 20 and 20,000 Hz; with the most important sounds in daily activities in the 250 to 6,000 Hz range. Speech includes a mix of low and high frequency sounds. Vowel sounds like "u" have low frequencies (250 to 1,000 Hz) and are usually easier to hear. Consonants like "s," "h," and "f," have higher frequencies (1,500 to 6,000 Hz) and are harder to hear. Consonants convey most of the meaning of what we say. Someone who cannot hear high-frequency sounds will have a hard time understanding speech. Intensity, or loudness, is measured in decibels (dB). A person with hearing within the normal range can hear sounds ranging from 0 to 140 dB. A whisper is around 30 dB. Conversations are usually 45 to 50 dB. Sounds that are louder than 90 dB can be uncomfortable to hear. A loud rock concert might be as loud as 110 dB. Sounds that are 120 dB or louder can be painful, and can result in temporary or permanent hearing loss.

Impairments in hearing can happen in either frequency or intensity, or both. Hearing loss severity is based on how well a person can hear the frequencies or intensities most often associated with speech. Severity can be described as mild, moderate, severe, or profound. The term "deaf" is sometimes used to describe someone who has an approximately 90 dB or greater hearing loss or who cannot use hearing to process speech and language information, even with the use of hearing aids. The term "hard of hearing" is sometimes used to describe people who have a less severe hearing loss than deafness.

Hearing loss can affect one or both ears and can be conductive, sensorineural, mixed or central. Approximately 30% of children who are deaf or hard of hearing also have one or more other developmental disabilities, such as intellectual disabilities, cerebral palsy, vision impairment, or epilepsy. Hearing loss can affect a child's ability to learn both to speak and to understand spoken language. This is especially true if the child is born with a hearing loss or loses his or her hearing before 2 years of age. People with hearing loss may communicate using speech (sometimes called oral communication), sign language (sometimes called manual communication), or a combination of both. Oral communication focuses on speech, listening with hearing aids, and sometimes lip reading. Manual communication includes sign language.

VISION IMPAIRMENT

The incidence, prevalence and causes of childhood vision impairment vary widely in different parts of the world depending up on the available health resources, general nutritional status and well-being, socioeconomic status, screening, and preventive practices. Vision impairment means that a person's eyesight cannot be corrected to a "normal" level. Vision impairment may be caused by a loss of visual acuity, where the eye does not see objects as clearly as usual. It may also be caused by a loss of visual field, where the eye cannot see as wide an area as usual without moving the eyes or turning the head. There are different ways of describing how severe a person's vision loss is. The World Health Organization defines "low vision" as visual acuity between 20/70 and 20/400, with the best possible correction, or a visual field of 20 degrees or less. "Blindness" is defined as a visual acuity worse than 20/400, with the best possible correction, or a visual field of 10 degrees or less. Someone with a visual acuity of 20/70 can see at 20 feet what someone with normal sight can see at 70 feet. Someone with a visual acuity of 20/400 can see at 20 feet what someone with normal sight can see at 400 feet. A normal visual field is about 160-170 degrees horizontally. Vision impairment severity may be categorized differently for certain purposes. In the United States, for example, the term "legal blindness" indicates that a person is eligible for certain education or federal programs. Legal blindness is defined as a visual acuity of 20/200 or worse, with the best possible correction, or a visual field of 20 degrees or less.

Visual acuity alone cannot tell you how much a person's life will be affected by their vision loss. It is important to also assess how well a person uses the vision they have. Two people may have the same visual acuity, but one may be able to use his or her vision better to do everyday tasks. Most people who are "blind" have at least some usable vision that can help them move around in their environment and do things in their daily lives. A person's functional vision can be evaluated by observing them in different settings to see how they use their vision. A functional vision evaluation can answer questions such as these: Can the person scan a room to find someone or something? What lighting is best for the person to do different tasks? How does the person use his or her vision to move around in a room or outside?

Vision impairment changes how a child understands and functions in the world. Impaired vision can affect a child's cognitive, emotional, neurological, and physical development by possibly limiting the range of experiences and the kinds of information a child is exposed to. Nearly two-thirds of children with vision impairment also have one or more other developmental disabilities, such as mental retardation, cerebral palsy, hearing loss, or epilepsy. Children with more severe vision impairment are more likely to have additional disabilities than are children with milder vision impairment.

CONCLUSION

Developmental disabilities or neurodevelopmental disabilities (includes intellectual disability) are a diverse group of chronic disorders that begin at any time during the development process (including conception, birth, and growth) up to 22 years of age and last throughout an individual's lifetime. The World Health Organization has developed the International Classification of Functioning, Disability, and Health (ICF) consists of three key components – body function and structure, activity, and participation – that provides a framework for delineating disabilities. The three key components of functioning and disability are inter-related and may interact with the health condition (e.g., disorder or disease) and personal and environmental factors. The reported prevalence of intellectual disability reflects consideration of the definition used, method of ascertainment of the data, and the characteristics of the population studied. Based on the typical bell shaped distribution of intelligence in the general population and 2 standard deviations below the mean as a cut off point, approximately 2.5% of the population is expected to have intellectual disability. Specific reading disability is fairly common, with up to 17.5% of children being affected. Centers for Disease Control and Prevention reports that the overall prevalence of ASDs in the United States is 9.0 per 1 000 population in children aged 8 years. The worldwide incidence of CP is estimated to be 2 to 3 per 1,000 live births. The prevalence of NTDs varies in different regions of the world. In the United States, the incidence of NTDs is 1 in 4 000 live births. The prevalence and causes of vision impairment vary in different parts of the world depending on multiple factors.

ACKNOWLEDGMENTS

This chapter is adapted with permission from authors' previous works: Patel DR, Merrick J. Intellectual disability, in Greydanus DE, Patel DR, Pratt HD, Calles J Jr, eds. Behavioral pediatrics, 3rd edition, New York: Nova Science, 2009:39-50; Patel DR, Greydanus DE, Calles J Jr, Pratt HD. Developmental disabilities across the life span. Disease a Month 2010;56(6):299-398. The sections on hearing loss and vision impairment are adapted from (public domain) United States Centers for Disease Control, http://www.cdc.gov/ncbddd/dd/ddhi.htm and http://www.cdc.gov/ncbddd/kids/vision.html accessed July 12, 2010.

REFERENCES

[1] Accardo PJ, ed. Cupute and Accardo's neurodevelopmental disabilities in infancy and childhood. 3rd edition, Volume 1 and 2. Baltimore, MD: Paul Brookes, 2008.

[2] World Health Organization. The international classification of functioning, disability, and health. Geneva: WHO, 2001.

[3] Cieza A, Stucki G. The International Classification of Functioning Disability and Health: its development process and content validity. Eur J Phys Rehabil Med 2008;44:303-13.

[4] The Individuals with Disabilities Education Improvement Act of 2004. 20 USC 1400 HR 1350 PL 108-446. URL: http://idea.ed.gov.

[5] The American with Disabilities Act. URL: http://www.ada.gov.

[6] What we mean by disability. URL: http://www.socialsecurity.gov.

[7] American Association of Intellectual and Developmental Disabilities. Intellectual disability: Definition, classification, and systems of sSupports. Washington, DC: Am Assoc Intellect Dev Disabil, 11th edition, 2010.

[8] Luckasson R, Borthwick-Duffy S, Buntix WHE, et al. Mental retardation: definition, classification, and system of supports. Washington, DC: Am Assoc Ment Retard, 10th edition, 2002.

[9] American Psychiatric Association. Diagnostic and statistical manual of mental disorders, 4th edition, Text Revision, Washington DC: Am Psychiatr Assoc, 2000:39-84.

[10] Walker WO, Johnson CP. Mental retardation: Overview and diagnosis. Pediatr Rev 2006;27(6):204-12.

[11] Shapiro BK, Batshaw M. Mental retardation (intellectual disability). In: Kliegman RM, Behrman RE, Jenson HB, Stanton BF, eds. Nelson Textbook of Pediatrics, 18th edition, Philadelphia: Elsevier Saunders, 2007:191-196.
[12] Intellectual disability. URL: http://www.cdc.gov/ncbddd/dd/mr3.htm
[13] McDermott S, Durkin MS, Schupf N, Stein ZA. Epidemiology and etiology of mental retardation. In: Jacobson JW, Mulick JA, Rojahn J, eds. Handbook of intellectual and developmental disabilities. New York: Springer, 2007:3-40.
[14] Yeargin-Allsopp M, Murphy CC, Cordero JF, Decouflé P, Hollowell JG. Reported biomedical causes and associated medical conditions for mental retardation among 10-year-old children, metropolitan Atlanta, 1985 to 1987. Dev Med Child Neurol 1997;39:142-9.
[15] Curry CJ, Stevenson RE, Anghton D, et al. Evaluation of mental retardation: recommendations of a consensus conference. Am J Med Genet 1997;72:468-77.
[16] Lagae L. Learning disabilities: definitions, epidemiology, diagnosis, and intervention strategies. Pediatr Clin North Am 2008;55(6):1259-1268.
[17] Shapiro B, Church RP, Lewis MEB. Specific learning disabilities. In: Batshaw ML, Pellegrino L, Roizen NJ, eds. Children with developmental disabilities. Baltimore, MD: Paul H Brookes, 6th edition, 2007:367-386.
[18] Shaywitz BA, Shaywitz SE. Dyslexia. Continuum 2001;8(5):17-36.
[19] Shaywitz SE, Shaywitz BA. Dyslexia (specific reading disability). Biol Psychiatry 2005;57:1301-9.
[20] Grizzle KL. Developmental dyslexia. Pediatr Clin North Am 2007;54:507-23.
[21] Shelley-Tremblay J, O'Brien N, Langhinrichsen-Rohling J. Reading disability in adjudicated youth: prevalence rates, current models, traditional and innovative treatments. Aggress Violent Behav 2007;12:376-92.
[22] Shalev RS. Dyscalculia. Continuum 2001;8:60-73.
[23] Shalev RS, Gross-Tsur V. Developmental dyscalculia. Pediatr Neurol 2001;24:334-42.
[24] Butterworth B. The development of arithmetical abilities. J Child Psychol Psychiatr 2005;46:3-18.
[25] Shalev RS, Manor O, Gross-Tsur V. Developmental dyscalculia: a prospective six-year follow-up. Dev Med Child Neurol 2005;47:121-5.
[26] Shalev RS, Auerbach J, Manor O, Gross-Tsur V. Developmental dyscalculia: prevalence and prognosis. Eur Child Adolesc Psychiatry 2000;9:58-64.
[27] Katusic SK, Colligan RC, Weaver AL, Barbaresi WJ. The forgotten learning disability: Epidemiology of written-language disorder in a population-based birth cohort (1976-1982), Rochester, Minnesota. Pediatrics 2009;123:1306-13.
[28] Deuel RK. Dysgraphia. Continuum 2001;8:37-59.
[29] Centers for Disease Control and Prevention. Prevalence of autism spectrum disorders – autism and developmental disabilities monitoring network, United States, 2006. MMWR 2009;58(SS 10):1-24.
[30] Autism spectrum disorders. URL: http://www.cdc.gov/ncbddd/autism.

[31] Rapin I, Tuchman RF. Autism: definition, neurobiology, screening, diagnosis. Pediatr Clin North Am 2008;55(5):1129-46.

[32] Wing L, Potter D. The epidemiology of autism spectrum disorders: Is the prevalence rising? MRDDRR 2002;8(3):151-61.

[33] Hughes JR. A review of recent reports on autism: 1000 studies published in 2007. Epilepsy Behav 2008;13:425-37.

[34] Matson JL, Shoemaker M. Intellectual disability and its relationship to autism spectrum disorders. Res Dev Disabil 2009;30:1107-14.

[35] de Bildt A, Sytema S, Kraijer D, Minderaa R. Prevalence of pervasive developmental disorders in children and adolescents with mental retardation. J Child Psychol Psychiatry 2005;46:275-86.

[36] Folstein SE. The clinical spectrum of autism. Clin Neurosci Res 2006;6:113-7.

[37] Battaglia A, Carey JC. Etiologic yield of autistic spectrum disorders: A prospective study. Am J Med Genet Part C 2006;142C:3-7.

[38] Cohen D, Pichard N, Tordjman S, Baumann C, Burglen L, Excoffier E, et al. Specific genetic disorders and autism: clinical contribution towards their identification. J Autism Dev Dis 2005;35:103-16.

[39] Cerebral palsy. URL: http://www.cdc.gov/ncbddd/dd/cp3.

[40] Paneth N. Establishing the diagnosis of cerebral palsy. Clin Obstetr Gynecol 2008;51(4):742-8.

[41] Horstmann HM, Bleck EE. Orthopaedic management in cerebral palsy, London: Mac Keith Press, 2nd edition, 2007:1-46,120-211.

[42] O'Shea TM. Cerebral palsy in very preterm infants: New epidemiological insights. Ment Retard Dev Disabl Res Rev 2002;8(3):135-45.

[43] Nelson KB. The epidemiology of cerebral palsy in term infants. Ment Retard Dev Disabl Res Rev 2002;8(3):146-50.

[44] Murphy N, Such-Neibar T. Cerebral palsy diagnosis and management: the state of the art. Curr Prob Pediatr Adolsce 2003;33(5):141-76.

[45] Ashwal S. Russman BS, Blasco PA, Miller G, Sandler A, Shevell M, Stevenson R. American Academy of Neurology Practice parameter: diagnostic assessment of the child with cerebral palsy. Neurology 2004;62:851-63.

[46] Dodge N. Cerebral palsy: Medical aspects. Pediatr Clin North Am 2008;55(5):1189-1208.

[47] Mitchell LE, Adzick NS, Melchionne J, Pasquariello PA, Sutton LN, Whitehead AS. Spina bifida. Lancet 2004;364:1885.

[48] Dias MS, Partington M. Embryology of myelomeningocele and enencephaly. Neurosurg Focus 2004;16(2):1-16.

[49] Liptak GS. Neural tube defects, In: Batshaw ML, Pellegrino L, Roizen NJ, eds. Children with developmental disabilities, Baltimore, MD: Paul H Brookes, 6th edition, 2007:419-38.

[50] Kerker BD, Owens PL, Zigler E, Horwitz SM. Mental health disorders among individuals with mental retardation: challenges to accurate prevalence estimates. Pub Health Rep 2004;119:409-17.

[51] Emerson E. Prevalence of psychiatric disorders in children and adolescents with and without intellectual disability. J Intellect Disabil Res 2003;47:51-8.

[52] Morgan VA, Leonard H, Bourke J, Jablensky A. Intellectual disability co-occurring with schizophrenia and other psychiatric illness: Population-based study. Br J Psychiatry 2008;193:364-72.

[53] Simonoff E, Pickles A, Charman T, Chandler S, Loucas T, Baird G. Psychiatric disorders in children with autism spectrum disorders: prevalence, comorbidity, and associated factors in a population-derived sample. J Am Acad Child Adolesc Psychiatry 2008;47:921-9.

[54] Hurtig T, Kuusikko S, Mattila M-L, Haapsamo H, Ebeling H, Jussila K, et al. Multi-informant reports of psychiatric symptoms among high-functioning adolescents with Asperger syndrome or autism. Autism 2009;13:583-98.

[55] Hofvander B, Delorme R, Chaste P, Nydén A, Wentz E, Ståhlberg O, et al. Psychiatric and psychosocial problems in adults with normal-intelligence autism spectrum disorders. BMC Psychiatry 2009;9:35.

SECTION ONE: INTELLECTUAL DISABILITY

In: Intellectual Disability
Editors: Ariel Tenenbaum et al.
ISBN: 978-1-53617-866-1

Chapter 2

A SYSTEMATIC LITERATURE REVIEW ON PEOPLE WITH INTELLECTUAL DISABILITY AND HEALTH

Mahfuz Ashraf**, PhD, Parves Sultan, PhD, Rashadul Hasan, Reema Harrison, PhD and Reece Hinchcliff, PhD

Entrepreneurship and Innovation, Crown Institute of Higher Education, Australia, School of Business and Law, Central Queensland University, Melbourne, Australia, Brainstorm Bangladesh, Dhaka, Bangladesh, School of Public Health and Community Medicine, UNSW Sydney, Australia and School of Public Health and Social Work, Faculty of Health, Queensland University of Technology, Sydney, Australia

* Corresponding Author: Mahfuz Ashraf, PhD, Crown Institute of Higher Education, 116 Pacific Highway North Sydney, NSW, Australia. E-mail: ashraf.mahfuz@gmail.com.

ABSTRACT

People with intellectual disability (ID) are vulnerable to poorer health outcomes than the general population, yet little is known about the optimal models for health promotion interventions for this population. This literature review was undertaken to identify the evidence base relating to health promotion for people with ID, the challenges experienced by this population and optimal approaches for intervention. Keywords, synonyms and subject headings relating to health promotion and ID were applied to eight electronic databases. Thirty-two studies met the inclusion criteria out of 7,390 research papers, and a narrative synthesis was undertaken to elicit key findings. Evidence to date suggests that the lack of theory-based interventions and an over-reliance on strategies that target cognitive beliefs are substantial challenges for developing effective interventions for the ID research. Whilst there is limited empirical evidence, the included studies suggest that tailored and theory-based interventions may be more successful in creating behavioural changes of the people with ID. The literature base is currently limited by a lack of comparable studies; making generalisations challenging. Greater theoretical and methodological justification to explain the personal, social, economic and behavioural drivers and consequences of health promotion interventions designed for people with ID are required.

INTRODUCTION

Health promotion is defined as 'the science and art of helping people change their lifestyle to move toward a state of optimal health' (1). In comparison to the general population, poor mental and physical health status is more common among people with intellectual disability (ID). According to the World Health Organization (WHO),

> "intellectual disability (ID) is a disorder defined by the presence of incomplete or arrested mental development, principally characterized by the deterioration of concrete functions at each stage of development and that contribute to the overall level of intelligence, such as cognitive, language, motor and socialization functions; in this anomaly, adaptation to the environment is always affected (2).

About 1–3 per cent of the world population is affected by diverse types of ID (3) and approximately 225 million people identify as having an ID worldwide (4). The number of people identifying as having an ID is increasing, yet knowledge of the policies and programs aimed at health promotion for people with ID is limited (5).

Both children and adults with ID are more susceptible to experiencing poorer health and often have poor health literacy (6). Health problems commonly identified in the ID population include inadequate physical activity, poor fitness, obesity, poor supply of nutrition or poor diet, cardiac disease, and poor knowledge of sexual health and contraceptives (7). Factors associated with such health concerns in the ID population are cognitive impairments, greater behavioural impairments, poorer living conditions and inadequate social networks (8). As such, developing health promotion interventions for people with ID is more complex than for the general population and requires careful consideration of the cognitive, affective and behavioural components (9).

The success of health promotion intervention is generally evaluated in terms of outcomes such as change in behaviour, self-management or self-efficacy (7). Self-management is one's ability to deal with one's own responsibility and emotional management to manage their own health condition (10), while self-efficacy is one's perceived confidence and ability to accomplish a recommended action (11). Depending on their condition, such outcomes may not be well-suited to those with an ID. Researchers have suggested different health promotion interventions and outcomes such as those that focus on changing and assessing skills (8). Therefore, the current research undertakes a systematic literature review process with particular emphasis on people with ID to: (i) identify evidence to date of health promotion activities, (ii) report the challenges in health promotion, and (iii) identify models for health promotion intervention and their successes.

OUR STUDY

A systematic literature review was undertaken in four phases: (a) Study search and selection process, (b) Relevance appraisal, (c) Data appraisal, and (d) Data extraction (12–14).

Table 1. Database searching summary

Searched database			**Number of articles found**		
Database	Field	Document Type	String 1	String 2	String 3
BMJ	All	All	7,534	407	32
EBSCOhost	Abstract	Articles	19,598	2,764	4
JSTOR	Abstract	Articles	9,542	2,712	354
ProQuest Central	Abstract	Articles	1,433,237	438,716	5,466
PubMed	Abstract	Articles	714,541	158,440	651
SAGE journals	Abstract	All	177,556	47,554	332
Springer	All	Articles	108,143	6,322	42
Wiley Online Library	Abstract	Journals	78,717	23,301	509
Total					7,390

Note:

[1] All the articles searched were published between the periods of 2010 to 2017.

[2] Articles searched using the search criteria read and download access.

Study search and selection process

Keywords, synonyms and subject headings relating to health promotion and ID were applied to eight electronic databases (BMJ, EBSCOhost, JSTOR, ProQuest Central, PubMed, SAGE Journals, Springer, and Wiley Online Library). Table 1 includes articles, published between January 2010 and August 2017. Search terms were developed based on the terms used in relevant published systematic reviews (15) and explored the indexing systems of the selected databases. The following combined search strings were applied to the eight electronic databases:

- String 1: (Health OR Healthcare)
- String 2: (Health OR Healthcare) AND (promotion OR education OR intervention OR program)
- String 3: (Health OR Healthcare) AND (promotion OR education OR intervention OR program) AND ('Intellectual disability'* OR 'Developmental disability'* OR 'Learning disability'* OR 'Mental disability'*)

Relevance appraisal

The search strategy returned a total of 7,390 potentially relevant articles. Both titles and abstracts were screened by two reviewers (R.H., M.A.), and full text articles retrieved for those considered relevant. Two reviewers then independently screened the full text articles against the inclusion and exclusion criteria based on the Population, Intervention, Comparison, Outcome (PICO) framework (16). The PICO framework helps to critically evaluate their relevance to the searched literature. The inclusion criteria were:

1) Population: Studies that explicitly include a sample with one or more intellectual disability (based on the WHO definition).
2) Intervention: Any health promotion intervention.
3) Comparison: None or a control group comparator.
4) Outcome: Any health promotion outcome including changes in health beliefs, intention or behaviour.

Exclusion criteria

Articles were excluded that did not focus on health promotion, did not provide outcome data for a population with an ID, duplicates, did not report primary data, were not published in English, not published between 2010-2017 or for which the full text was not available. A total of 4,921 articles were excluded for not considering people with ID and health promotion as focal study point (see Figure 1).

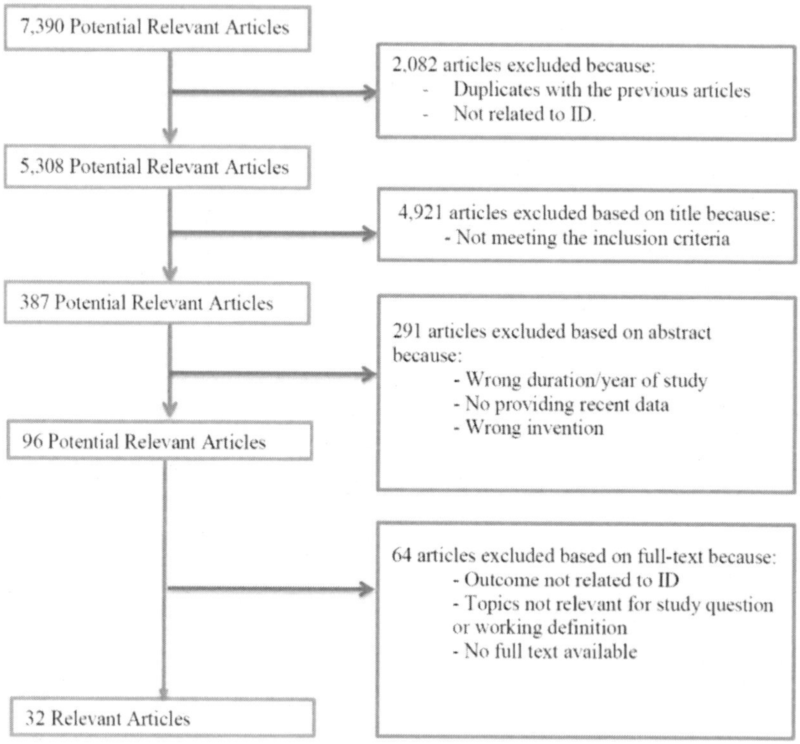

Figure 1. Steps in the inclusion and exclusion criteria.

Data appraisal

For each included article, reviewers independently applied four quality appraisal criteria adapted from Popay's (17) rating scale (scoring as, 0=weak, 1=moderate, 2=strong for each criterion) for evaluating the risk of bias in the data.

1) Aims and objectives are clearly stated
2) Clear description of study context

3) Description of the intervention is present
4) Inclusion of sufficient data for evidence and interpretation

The four-point tool was developed where the papers which score five or more was as good, a score of 3 to 4 rated as being of moderate quality, and studies scoring two or less were rated poor. Our 32 studies were passed through this data appraisal process (see Figure 1).

Data Extraction and Synthesis

A thematic analysis was conducted to find the studies of health promotion and identify key themes in relation to the research objectives. For the thematic analysis, three steps were followed (18): 1) coding of text 'line-by-line'; 2) the development of 'descriptive themes'; and 3) analytic exploration of the themes. In the step of coding of text 'line-by-line', the findings of primary studies were organised based on 'free codes' related to the research objectives. Three authors individually coded each line of verbatim findings according to its meaning and content using NVivo (version 11) (19). Each sentence/line derived from the studies was given at least one code, however, most were tagged with multiple codes. Then, these initial codes were categorised to group under descriptive themes. An analytic approach was taken to explore these descriptive themes in relation to the review questions.

FINDINGS

In total, 32 studies (see Figure 1) met the inclusion criteria. Twenty-three codes were identified in initial coding of text ‘line-by-line’ resulting in ‘descriptive themes’. These themes were assessed in relation to the research objectives. Table 2 shows the key themes and relevant discussions.

Table 2. Summarisation of findings according to the key themes

Key themes	Key points in the discussion
Challenges for health promotion amongst people with ID	1) Lack of understanding of different levels of awareness of the people with ID is critical to overcome the barriers in successful health promotion programs (22). 2) Motivating the people with ID for paying attention to the objectives of a health promotion is challenging in health promotion process (21). 3) Health promotion materials should be developed considering difficulties with memory, concentration, consequential thinking, planning, and lower ability to apply abstract knowledge of people with ID (20). 4) Low educational level of staff working in people with ID has been identified as a barrier to get maximum benefits of health promotion (23). 5) Due to the cognitive impairment associated with ID, a combined approach is necessary with a more comprehensive health behaviour education programme for people with ID (22). 6) Consideration of the preferences of people with ID improves the drive to adhere with the message and instructions of health promotion (6). 7) Including people with ID in the process of developing health promotion materials is important to get maximum benefits of health promotion (26).
Models for intervention	1) While promoting assistive technology (AT), the promoters should consider the flexibility, and different levels of inability of people with ID (20). 2) Today, there are many emerging ideas in the landscape of health promotion research, most of these are tailored in nature (6). 3) The perceptions and prior knowledge of the people without ID are also important while developing health promotion materials (8). 4) Theory-based interventions are found to be evidently useful, that can also be used in multiple contexts (5). 5) Peer support in group-based intervention is found to be useful while encouraging behavioural changes (20) 6) Theory-based health promotion intervention allows in reproducing similar effectiveness in intervention outcome while understanding the cause of specific behaviour changes (24). 7) Finding a sound methodology is a big research challenge for health promotions research for the people with ID (26). 8) Further research is needed into multi-disciplinary programmes which incorporate the primary carers and are responsive to NICE guidelines (27). 9) It is important to understand the preferences, perceptions and barriers of the people with ID beforehand while choosing the type of intervention (28). 10) The effectiveness of health promotion intervention is evaluated considering the individual, institutional, home-group and community settings (7).

Key themes	Key points in the discussion
	11) Future studies need to include occupational perspectives and social determinants (e.g., specific context and needs etc.) in ID related studies (29). 12) Group-based educational intervention is found to be more effective in terms of long-term health benefits than curricula-based intervention (25). 13) Intervention with consecutive follow-up for longer period helps in adherence over time by people with ID (25). 14) It is also important to follow a flexible, self-reporting and participatory approach while implementing a multi-component intervention effectively (6). 15) The effective health promotion interventions need to influence at multiple levels by focusing not only changing health behaviour of people with ID (29). 16) Need to examine how health promotion programs may be adapted to be meaningful for people with more severe disabilities (26). 17) There is a need for tailored and specific health promotion approach for people with ID (5). 18) Today, there are many emerging ideas and themes which is increasing the landscape of health promotion research. Most of these ideas are tailored in nature (6). 19) The health promotors now need to provide knowledge about exercise, nutritional facts, community-based activities and peer supports (22). 20) If specific and specialised health promotion approach are not followed, the health information in the health promotion would not be passed adequately for preventing health issues (30). 21) There is a need for tailored and specific health promotion approach to address the risks of primary and secondary disease for this target group (5). 22) While exchanging health information with different people with ID, it is important to follow individualised approach (30). 23) Existing health promotion programmes for people with ID must be tailored to individual preferences and motivations (31). 24) A tailored health promotional strategy for older people with ID should consider the domain of assistive technology, recreational activities, and diet (5). 25) While promoting assistive technology (AT), the promoters should consider the flexibility and, as well as, different levels of inability of people with ID (20). 26) Without specific and specialised health promotion approach, there would be inadequate health information exchange between people with ID (30). 27) There is a need for support from both from the governmental and private welfare services, and as well as, services from volunteer organisations, family members or relatives in developing health promotion strategies for people with ID (5). 28) There is a need for holistic involvement in designing health promotion interventions (32).

Table 2. (Continued)

Key themes	Key points in the discussion
	29) As children are usually not capable to adhere to a well-designed intervention, in such cases, training to the parents helps more to the children to adhere to a designed intervention (33). 30) The most appropriate means of engaging care givers in a way that will reliably impact on health outcomes of the people with ID remains, as yet, unknown (33). 31) Health promotion and disease prevention strategies for older people with ID should be modified to the individuals' health status, social needs and abilities, and psychological concerns (5). 32) Areas of intervention should include mental and physical health, housing, work opportunities, adapted AT, physical exercises, recreational activities, leisure time, and diet monitoring (5).

Challenges of health promotion for people with ID

Five key considerations emerged from this theme. Firstly, the need to consider difficulties often experienced and associated with memory, concentration, consequential thinking, planning, and ability to apply abstract knowledge (20). The use of pictures and visual aids, simple language, and clearly articulated and repeated instructions in intervention materials may all assist in ensuring the intervention is well-explained and adhered to.

Although people with ID are often discussed as homogenous population, ID describes a broad range of types and levels of impairment which may require a range of different adaptations in order to develop suitable intervention materials (6). It is challenging to provide a range of accessible formats of health promotion materials that address the different levels and types of capacity of people with ID. Related to this, some people with ID have lower levels of health literacy, and therefore, it is important to understand the knowledge and potential intervention of participants before engaging in health promotion efforts (21). For example, it has been reported that women with ID may have less awareness and knowledge regarding sexual health, therefore, an intervention to increase the use of contraceptive products may require baseline assessment of existing knowledge and then a tailored educational component that accounts for this (7).

Many health promotion efforts utilise social support to engage participants and maintain their motivation. Lack of social support is often associated with the older population with ID, which poses a challenge for such an approach (22). In order to ensure active engagement in the health promotion process, consideration of the characteristics of the intervention group, their preferences, skills, and self-efficacy are important to ensure an appropriate intervention strategy (23). Finally, Elinder et al. (23) highlighted that a lack of knowledge amongst staff or home caregivers working in people with ID about health promotion can creates further difficulties when attempting to undertake an intervention as they may not effectively facilitate engagement in the intervention effort.

Models for health promotion intervention for this population and their success

Sixteen studies discussed evidence-based intervention models for people with ID (see Table 2). The included studies highlighted that current models for health promotion intervention lack sufficient emphasis on the social and environmental context on which people with ID often depend to make their choices and actions (8). Heller et al. (6) in 2014 propose, five strategies or developing suitable health promotion interventions for people with ID: 1) using theory-based intervention; 2) use of group-based strategies that include peer learning and engagement 3) scientific research design; 4) inclusion of local context; 5) greater focus on conditions related to health or society (6).

Three of these approaches were discussed in the included literature. Firstly, the use of theory-based interventions enables researchers to not only test an intervention but also to understand the underlying mechanisms that cause specific behavioural changes (24). This is critical in the context of the diverse intervention aims and participant groups that are under the umbrella of health promotion interventions for people with ID.

Secondly, the use of a group-based educational intervention was reported to be more effective than curricula-based intervention in terms of long-term health benefits within the family and community (25). Such intervention with consecutive follow-up for longer period helps in adherence over time by people with ID. Likewise, peer support intervention is found to be useful while encouraging behavioural changes (20).

A scientific research design includes a multi-component intervention model and considers the intervention characteristics, types of individual commitments, organizational capacity and societal aspects (6). Approaches that utilise a flexible, self-reporting and participatory approach, with an extensive preparation phase may facilitate participant engagement.

Finally, studies highlight the need to consider the specific condition and participant group in order to develop an effective intervention approach. For example, behaviour-based health promotion interventions and psycho-social interventions, were reported as beneficial for improving physical activity, cognitive function and self-management behaviours in older people with ID with chronic conditions (26). A pragmatic approach to effective interventions addressing issues, such as excessive obesity and the related clinical and financial issues amongst people with ID were considered effective (27). Curtin (28) in 2015 highlighted the importance of understanding the preferences, perceptions and barriers of the ID population being targeted when developing the intervention. Health promotion interventions were generally likely to have greater success not only to change health behaviour, but also to address the dynamic social factors surrounding an individual, in addition to the individual's own behaviour (29).

The included studies report that developing tailored health promotion approaches makes the health promotion more meaningful, and this is because of the diversity of impairments amongst people with ID. Tailored interventions should consider broader domains of health promotion, such as cognitive ability, mental and physical health, living place and workplace considerations. A first step towards tailoring health promotion initiative is to ensure more inclusive participation and use involvement in design. The use of a specific theoretical approach, such as 'social cognitive theory', for example, may be very useful in conveying health information for preventing tobacco and alcohol use among the people with mild to moderate IDs, but this theoretical approach may not be suitable for those with severe IDs or for those with particular conditions (20). Therefore, research argues for a need of tailored and specific health promotion approaches and frameworks to address any given target group (5, 30, 31).

When included in interventions for the general population, people with ID do not get the same benefits as people without ID. Co-creating health promotion materials specifically for the given target group is one strategy to ensure that a suitable intervention is developed (26). In developing health promotion strategies for people with ID, support may also be required from support persons, carers, government and private health and welfare services, family members and relatives (5). There is a need for holistic approach in designing health promotion interventions (32), and this may be possible by engaging both healthcare staff and people with ID when designing health promotion interventions. This can further be extended by involving and providing appropriate educational resources and lifestyle skill training to the parents of children with specific ID, such as excessive food consumption (33).

DISCUSSION

Current research on people with ID is mostly dominated by meta-analysis, and thus, qualitative in nature. While the findings above show concerns about the challenges of health promotion intervention, effectiveness and involvement, there is a lack of sound methodology to be followed to conduct study on people with ID (26). Before undertaking any study on the people with ID, it is often challenging to identify and employ the right methodology and theory to explain personal, social, economic and behavioural circumstances and factors of people with ID, and particularly the factors that moderate and mediate the causal factors and outcomes of any health promotion. Therefore, research collaboration among cognate disciplines may provide sound and comprehensive findings in the field of health promotion and intervention of intellectual disability.

There is no adequate evidence to suggest that any particular model is better than another type of intervention design. For example, as children are usually not capable to adhere to a well-designed intervention, in such cases, training to the parents helps more to their ID children to adhere to objectives of a health promotion intervention. The effectiveness of health promotion intervention is evaluated by considering the individual, institutional, home-group and community settings. As both men and women with IDs have limited health literacy, cognitive inability and incapacity in physical developmental, understanding the complexity of their needs and all the influencing factors that affect their health and wellbeing status are significant in the process of implementing effective health promotion strategies (7).

The current studies in the literature recommend for the necessity of health promotion studies with particular emphasis on people with ID. These include: how gender (7), age (i.e., gerontological study) (6), care-givers' skills (8, 27), obesity (34), genetic/biological difference (35), and inter-rater reliability (36) influence the physical, mental and social activities of people with ID.

One of the major challenges to direct research on people with ID is the data collection protocol and ethical issues. There are general guidelines on how to clearly state and inform the risk, terms and conditions to the subjects (people with ID) while seeking consent for recruiting them in study. While recruitment must be fully voluntary and free from coercion (37), data collection with people with ID could be challenging with the observational and ethnographic methods to gain insights about the participants' lifestyle, or exploring and connecting the meaning of observed activities (38). As the presence of multiple group members increase the interaction between people with ID and as well as provide adequate time to ask and share experience and views with each other (37), multiple focus groups and large samples are useful means to identify and explore diverse perspectives of health promotions for the people with ID (39, 40). Besides, access and adequacy of enough samples/subjects remain another challenge to ID research, which many potentially lead to lack of robust evidence-based studies to measure the health promotion outcomes for the people with ID (9).

While developing health promotion for people with ID, Cardell (29) in the 2015 study suggested to include the occupational perspectives (e.g., doing, becoming, achieving something) and social determinants (e.g., specific context and needs etc.) in ID related studies. This is because people with ID are more susceptible to engage in activities, and thus, an occupational perspective for people with ID needs to be considered to overcome any physical, social, political and economic constraints. However, these issues are inadequate in literature to date (38).

There is also a lack of a valid and reliable scale to appropriately measure the outcomes and effects of any health promotion intervention, in general. In this connection, a number of studies concluded that there is a lack of sound theories explaining appropriate methodology to identify the causal factors and outcome of health promotion intervention for the people with ID (8, 26). While research on people with ID can be time consuming and budget dependant, a methodology following social science perspective can add value to the health promotion research in ID.

The aim of this study was to explore the pattern findings from the current studies on health promotion for ID people and to identify the critical issues addressed in current literature. This study shows that research on health promotion intervention for people with ID have been increasing over the last few years, however, little research is undertaken on designing and evaluating theory-based health promotion and measuring behavioural change using explicit techniques. The review also revealed that most of the studies were qualitative, with a few are well-designed experimental studies. Besides, there is a lack of study on health promotion intervention evaluating the outcomes of the Assistive Technology designed for people with ID.

Overall, the review of literature highlights that there is a clear lack of enough studies in various contexts and cultural backgrounds to explain how and why certain intervention works, which of the data collection techniques are useful and in what specific contexts, what theoretical consideration can better explain the personal, social, economic and behavioural consequences of health promotion intervention for people with ID, how technology mediated intervention works and how effective these are, what techniques are useful to collect large sample sizes for both qualitative and quantitative research methods, and finally, whether cross-sectional, longitudinal, or comparative studies in various contexts can effectively produce ID research outcomes. To effectively compare and measure the outcomes of health promotion interventions for people with ID, future studies should also follow theory-based frameworks to study techniques in different cultural and geographic contexts.

CONCLUSION

This review was designed as a preliminary foundation of current research relating to health promotion for intellectually disable (ID) people. One of the major limitations of this study is that this review has not included any discussion of "intervention period" and "intervention origin." However, it is expected that future work would benefit from the findings of this study. A further development of search criteria, inclusion of more research database and stricter inclusion criteria could further improve the findings of this study.

REFERENCES

[1] O'Donnell MP. Definition of health promotion. Am J Health Promot 1986;1(1):4-5.

[2] Katz G, Lazcano-Ponce E. Intellectual disability: definition, etiological factors, classification, diagnosis, treatment and prognosis. Salud Publica Mex 2008;50:132-41.

[3] Riazuddin S, Hussain M, Razzaq A, Iqbal Z, Shahzad M, Polla DL, et al. Exome sequencing of Pakistani consanguineous families identifies 30 novel candidate genes for recessive intellectual disability. Mol Psychiatry 2017;22(11):16-22.

[4] Ndengeyingoma A, Ruel J. Nurses' representations of caring for intellectually disabled patients and perceived needs to ensure quality care. J Clin Nurs 2016;25(21-22):3199-3208.

[5] Carmeli E, Imam B. Health promotion and disease prevention strategies in older adults with intellectual and developmental disabilities. Front Public Health 2014;2:31.

[6] Heller T, Fisher D, Marks B, Hsieh K. Interventions to promote health: crossing networks of intellectual and developmental disabilities and aging. Disabil Health J 2014;7(1):24-32.

[7] Bollard M. Health promotion and intellectual disability: listening to men. Health Soc Care Commun 2017;25(1):185-93.

[8] Naaldenberg J, Kuijken N, van Dooren K, de Valk HV. Topics, methods and challenges in health promotion for people with intellectual disabilities: A structured review of literature. Res Dev Disabil 2013;34(12):34-45.

[9] Cooray S, Bhaumik S, Michael DM, Torales J, Ng R, Ventriglio A. Health promotion in people with intellectual disabilities. Int J Culture Ment Health 2016;9(4):430-53.

[10] McCorkle R, Ercolano E, Lazenby M, Schulman-Green D, Schilling LS, Lorig K, et al. Self-management: Enabling and empowering patients living with cancer as a chronic illness. CA Cancer J Clin 2011;61(1):50-62.

[11] Green EC, Murphy E. Health belief model. In: The Wiley Blackwell encyclopedia of health, illness, behavior and society. Chichester: John Wiley, 2014:766-69.

[12] Moher D, Liberati A, Tetzlaff J, Altman DG, Prisma Group. Preferred reporting items for systematic reviews and meta-analyses: The PRISMA statement. PLoS Med 2009;6(7):e1000097.

[13] Chiarini G, Ray P, Akter S, Masella C, Ganz A. mHealth technologies for chronic diseases and elders: A systematic review. IEEE J Select Areas Communications 2013;31(9):6-18.

[14] Racine M, Tousignant-Laflamme Y, Kloda LA, Dion D, Dupuis G, Choinière M. A systematic literature review of 10 years of research on sex/gender and experimental pain perception–Part 1: Are there really differences between women and men? Pain 2012;153(3):602-18.

[15] Roy MJ, Donaldson C, Baker R, Kerr S. The impacts of social enterprise-led activity on health and well-being: an integrative review. Prospero Int Prospect Register Syst Rev 2012;4(2):1–6.

[16] Mosa AS, Yoo I, Sheets L. A systematic review of healthcare applications for smartphones. BMC Med Inform Decis Mak 2012;12:67.

[17] Rodgers M, Sowden A, Petticrew M, Arai L, Roberts H, Britten N, et al. Testing methodological guidance on the conduct of narrative synthesis in systematic reviews: effectiveness of interventions to promote smoke alarm ownership and function. Evaluation 2009;15(1):49-73.

[18] Thomas J, Harden A. Methods for the thematic synthesis of qualitative research in systematic reviews. BMC Med Res Methodol 2008;8:39-45.

[19] Ashraf MM, Hasan N, Lewis L, Hasan MR, Ray P. A systematic literature review of the application of information communication technology for visually impaired people. Int J Disabil Manage 2016;16(1):1-11.

[20] Kerr S, Lawrence M, Middleton AR, Fitzsimmons L, Darbyshire C. Tobacco and alcohol use in people with mild/moderate intellectual disabilities: Giving voice to their health promotion needs. J Appl Res Intellect Disabil 2017;30(4):612-26.

[21] Sundblom E, Bergström H, Ellinder LS. Understanding the implementation process of a multi-component health promotion intervention for adults with intellectual disabilities in Sweden. J Appl Res Intellect Disabil 2015;28(4):296-306.

[22] Doody CM, Doody O. Health promotion for people with intellectual disability and obesity. Br J Nurs 2012;21(8):460-5.

[23] Elinder LS, Bergström H, Hagberg J, Wihlman U, Hagströmer M. Promoting a healthy diet and physical activity in adults with intellectual disabilities living in community residences: Design and evaluation of a cluster-randomized intervention. BMC Public Health 2010;10(1):761-9.

[24] Van Schijndel-Speet M, Evenhuis HM, van Empelen P, van Wijck R, Echteld MA. Development and evaluation of a structured programme for promoting physical activity among seniors with intellectual disabilities: a study protocol for a cluster randomized trial. BMC Public Health 2013;13(1):746-56.

[25] Heller T, McCubbin JA, Drum C, Peterson J. Physical activity and nutrition health promotion interventions: what is working for people with intellectual disabilities? Intellect Dev Disabil 2011;49(1):26-36.

[26] Scott HM, Havercamp SM. Systematic review of health promotion programs focused on behavioral changes for people with intellectual disability. Intellect Dev Disabil 2016;54(1):63-76.

[27] Thomas GR, Kerr MP. Longitudinal follow-up of weight change in the context of a community-based health promotion programme for adults with an intellectual disability. J App Res Intellect Disabil 2011;24(4):381-7.

[28] Curtin C, Bandini LG, Must A, Phillips S, Maslin MC, Lo C, et al. Including youth with intellectual disabilities in health promotion research: Development and reliability of a structured interview to assess the correlates of physical activity among youth. J Appl Res Intellect Disabil 2016;29(4):378-86.

[29] Cardell B. Reframing health promotion for people with intellectual disabilities. Global Qual Nurs Res 2015;10(2):233-305.

[30] Mastebroek M, Naaldenberg J, van den Driessen Mareeuw FA, Leusink GL, Lagro-Janssen AL, van Schrojenstein Lantman-de HM. Health information exchange for patients with intellectual disabilities: a general practice perspective. Br J Gen Pract 2016; 66(1):720-8.

[31] Kuijken NM, Naaldenberg J, Nijhuis-van der Sanden MW, Schrojenstein-Lantman de Valk HM. Healthy living according to adults with intellectual disabilities: towards tailoring health promotion initiatives. J Intellect Disabil Res 2016 60(3):228-41.

[32] Hanna LM, Taggart L, Cousins W. Cancer prevention and health promotion for people with intellectual disabilities: An exploratory study of staff knowledge. J Intellect Disabil Res 2011;55(3):281-91.

[33] Hithersay R, Strydom A, Moulster G, Buszewicz M. Carer-led health interventions to monitor, promote and improve the health of adults with intellectual disabilities in the community: a systematic review. Res Dev Disabil 2014;35(4):887-907.

[34] Krause S, Ware R, McPherson L, Lennox N, O'Callaghan M. Obesity in adolescents with intellectual disability: Prevalence and associated characteristics. Obes Res Clin Pract 2016;10(5):520-30.

[35] Van Wijngaarden-Cremers PJ, van Eeten E, Groen WB, Van Deurzen PA, Oosterling IJ, Van der Gaag RJ. Gender and age differences in the core triad of impairments in autism spectrum disorders: a systematic review and meta-analysis. J Autism Dev Disord 2014; 44(3):627-35.

[36] Horner-Johnson W, Bailey D. Assessing understanding and obtaining consent from adults with intellectual disabilities for a health promotion study. J Policy Pract Intellect Disabil 2013;10(3):260-5.

[37] Swaine J, Parish SL, Luken K, Atkins L. Recruitment and consent of women with intellectual disabilities in a randomised control trial of a health promotion intervention. J Intellect Disabil Res 2011;55(5):474-83.

[38] Channon A. Intellectual disability and activity engagement: Exploring the literature from an occupational perspective. J Occupat Sci 2014;21(4):443-58.

[39] Paton C, Bhatti S, Purandare K, Roy A, Barnes TR. Quality of prescribing of antipsychotic medication for people with intellectual disability under the care of UK mental health services: A cross-sectional audit of clinical practice. BMJ Open 2016;6(12):131-9.

[40] Hubbard KL, Bandini LG, Folta SC, Wansink B, Must A. The adaptation of a school-based health promotion programme for youth with intellectual and developmental disabilities: A community-engaged research process. J Appl Res Intellect Disabil 2014;27(6):576-90.

In: Intellectual Disability
Editors: Ariel Tenenbaum et al.
ISBN: 978-1-53617-866-1

Chapter 3

PREVALENCE RATE OF INTELLECTUAL DISABILITY AMONG CHILDREN IN BARWANI, INDIA

Ram Lakhan**, *DrPH and Anthony Mawson, MA, DrPH
Department of Epidemiology and Biostatistics,
School of Public Health Initiative, Jackson State University,
Medical Mall, Jackson, Mississippi, United States of America

ABSTRACT

Intellectual disability (ID) is a global public health concern. Although developed countries have well-established systems for identifying persons with ID and providing services, this is not the case in many low and middle income (LAMI) countries, including India. In order to help the Indian government to plan for health care, education, employment and welfare service needs, a cross-sectional study aimed at determining the prevalence of ID in children ages 3-18 years was carried out in District

* Corresponding Author: Ram Lakhan, DrPH, Department of Epidemiology and Biostatistics, School of Public Health Initiative, Jackson State University, 350 W Woodrow Wilson Drive, Suite 320, Medical Mall, Jackson, MS 39213-7681, United States. E-mail: ramlakhan@gmail.com.

Barwani, state of Madhya Pradesh, India, representing both a tribal and non-tribal population. Community-based rehabilitation workers administered a standard screening checklist. The Developmental Screening Test and Vineland Social Maturity Scale were administered to identified cases to determine their level of ID. The prevalence rate (percent) of ID was 5.67 (95% CI: 4.24, 7.10) in tribal populations and 3.11 (95% CI: 2.03, 4.19) among non-tribal groups. Prevalence rates of ID were higher in younger age-groups (3-6 years, 1.42/1000) than in older children (15-18 years, 0.54/1000). The prevalence of ID was 83% higher in the tribal population than in the non-tribal groups (OR = 1.83; 95% CI: 1.42, 2.32) but did not differ by gender (OR = 1.05; 95% CI: 0.826, 1.344).

INTRODUCTION

Intellectual disability (ID) is a global public health concern. Estimates of the prevalence of ID are needed to plan for health care, education, employment, welfare and other special services. Unlike developed countries such as the United States (US), which have well established systems for identifying and providing services for people with ID, the Indian government does not have a systematic approach to identifying children with ID (1-2). Although this is not the case in low and middle income (LAMI) countries such as India, which has the second largest population in the world, but lacks data on the national prevalence of ID (1-2). Because of this lacuna, many people with ID in India remain unidentified and therefore unable to receive the available health and social services (3). In general, LAMI countries have higher prevalence rates of disability than developed nations (4).

The prevalence of ID is uncertain, because population-based studies have not been undertaken in India (1). This presents a problem for planners and the organizations that seek to provide services for people and communities with ID. Epidemiologic studies assess the magnitude of the problem and plan appropriately for the resources needed (1). The lack of such studies in India poses challenges for the organizations assisting people with ID. The most recent government survey that included ID for the first time lacked proper ID definition and methodology (5). Non-trained enumerators also conducted the survey, in which people with chronic mental illness were conflated with ID because some had a mental disability.

India has a very diverse population. According to the Statistical Profile of Scheduled Tribes in India (SPSTI), a report of Ministry of tribal Affairs, Tribal (Adivasi) populations, commonly categorized under schedule tribal/caste, account for 8.6% of the total population of the country (6) but remain unaccounted for in all ID surveys, reports and studies. This group is not only deprived in health care, education, and employment, but also in practicing their religion, culture and in many other ways (6-7). The tribal population occupies the lowest and poorest section of the national social hierarchy. The term Adivasi is often used as a synonym for backwardness, illiteracy, and even with mental illness, by the mainstream population. Tribal groups live in 13 states of the country, but over half are concentrated in the six states of Madhya Pradesh (14.51%), Maharashtra (10.17%), Orissa (9.66%), Gujarat (8.87%), Rajasthan (8.42%) and Jharkhand (8.4%) (SPSTI, 2013).

Within the tribal population there are 47 groups, many speaking different languages. Most of the groups live in remote forests or other isolated, geographically difficult terrains, with few connections to modern life (7). Their traditions and cultural practices also differ from those of the majority population groups, comprising Hindu, Muslims, Sikh, and Christians. Polygamy, consanguineous marriage, marriage at very early age for girls, and traditional use of alcohol on occasion of death, marriage and birth in both genders male and female, are widely practiced. The traditional alcoholic drink is prepared through the distillation process from Mahua (Hindi name) flower (*Madhuca longifolia*).

The Tribal population has a high prevalence of nutritional disorders, infectious diseases such as dysentery, tuberculosis, malaria, and genetic disorders related to red blood cells such as sickle cell disease. Health remains very poor in tribal populations across the country because of their preference for traditional health care that is mainly based on the use of herbs, plants, and faith healing. Poor awareness of health issues, poor health infrastructure in rural tribal areas, lack of transportation, poverty, and the lack of willingness of medical professionals to serve in these communities are other important factors that contribute to the poor health conditions of the tribal population (7-9).

Worldwide, the prevalence of ID is estimated at 1-4% (10). The point prevalence of ID in India ranges from 1 to 32 per 1000, depending upon case definition and methodology used in the studies (11). Most of the studies conducted in India used ICD-10 criteria of ID, which have shown huge variation in prevalence rates. In rural communities, the prevalence of ID (IQ < 50) was found to be 3.4 per 1000 (12). In another study, it was 34.2 per 1000 for severe intellectual disability (IQ < 35) (13). Prevalence rates reported in India vary immensely. It is likely that the National Sample Survey Organization (NSSO) data do not reflect the full extent of disability in India (3, 14). Considering all of these factors, a cross-sectional study is needed to provide an improved estimate of the prevalence of ID in tribal and non-tribal population.

Services for people with ID in the State of Madhya Pradesh are very limited. There are very few rehabilitation organizations located in resource-poor areas that provide services to the rural population. Ashagram Trust (AGT) is a nonprofit organization started in 1983 for the rehabilitation of people with leprosy, situated in Barwani. This organization started a community-based rehabilitation project with financial help from Action Aid for people with disabilities in Barwani block. The organization obtained disability data from government departments but the data were inaccurate and outdated. The Community-Based Rehabilitation (CBR) team and its funding partner needed a precise estimate of the number of ID people living in the project area. The present study was planned and conducted for that purpose. A previous study conducted using a mixed-method approach covered only four villages with a 99% tribal population (15), but the project had an almost 60% non-tribal population, so that the results were not representative of the project population. The non-tribal population has relatively better living conditions and facilities related to education, health, sanitation, employment and transportation. Even so, approximately 77% of the population lives in poverty. Both populations are highly varied in their culture, practices, and beliefs.

Community based rehabilitation currently provides rehabilitation services for people with disabilities (16). It was proposed by the World Health Organization (WHO) as the most appropriate model of rehabilitation in poor communities. Other researchers have also found it useful due to its cultural sensitivity, accessibility and cost-effectiveness in India (9).

In this research, we used ICD-10-based criteria to classify people with ID according to their IQ level, as this is the most widely used classification system across all member countries of WHO (1, 17). This system classifies people with ID into the categories of: Borderline ID (IQ > 70), Mild ID (IQ 50-69), Moderate ID (IQ 35-49), Severe ID (IQ 20-34) and Profound ID (IQ < 20). The definition of intellectual disability proposed by Grossman (1983) was based on three components -- 1) significant sub-average intelligence, 2) concurrent impairment in adaptive behavior, and 3) occurrence during development – and was used to explain ID to parents and the community during the survey (18).

The objective in this paper was to estimate the prevalence of ID in children ages 3 to 18 years in Barwani block of Barwani District in Madhya Pradesh state, India and to conduct a cross-sectional survey to identify people with ID under a community-based rehabilitation project in Barwani.

OUR STUDY

The project covered 63 villages of Barwani block, comprising tribal and non-tribal groups. Only 51 villages with the current population of 63,789 (males – 32,759 and females – 31,030) were covered in this study, because at the beginning of the project the 12 remaining villages were facing political unrest due to a popular movement to oppose "Sardar Sarover dam" on the Narmada river (Narvada Bachao Andolan). Among the study villages, the total tribal population was 24,681 persons (males 12,575;

females 12,106) and the non-tribal population was 39,108 (males 20,184; females 18,924) (19). Barwani district is one of the poorest districts in India (15). The overall composition of the population of this district is 68% tribal and 32% non-tribal (19), but this ratio is almost opposite in Barwani block, where the tribal population comprises about 40% of the total population, of which about 53% live below the poverty line. The tribal population is the most disadvantaged in the district (9).

Research instrument and testing. The "National Institute for the Mentally Handicapped Developmental Screening Schedule (NIMH-DDS)" is a valid and reliable tool available in India (20), although, there is little evidence of its use in the community, probably because of the absence of community-based studies in the country. Even in government surveys, however, family members are asked to name persons in the household with ID, which assumes that family members are aware of ID (5). NIMH-DDS was developed by Madhavan, Menon, Kalyan, Narayan and Subbarao (1988) at the National Institute for the Mentally Handicapped (NIMH) India (21). The tool was specifically designed for use by Community-Based Rehabilitation Workers (CBRWs).

Ashagram Trust had the tool translated into the Hindi language for use in this project. This tool was also used in earlier tribal population research project and was found to be sensitive and suitable instrument for use (15). CBRWs involved in the survey received one week of training on various aspects of ID, CBR and on this tool by the CBR team. The team leaders included a psychiatrist, a clinical psychologist, and two specialists in intellectual disabilities. Four CBRWs with previous experience in conducting this kind of survey were also involved in the data collection process. CBRWs visited door-to-door and were supervised by specialists in intellectual disabilities. "Sarpanch" is an elected position in village. Sarpanch supervise and monitor all development work in their village. Consent from Sarpanches (as they are collectively called) to conduct the survey was obtained by organizing an event at the Ashagram head quarter (Rain Basera). All Sarpanches of those villages were invited and were asked to support the project. Informed consent was obtained from the householders during the survey.

Estimation of socio-economic status was difficult due to non-availability of a suitable scale for assessing the mixed population at that time. Specifically, it was noted that the tribal population had so little information about numbers that they counted money on the scale of twenty. For example, if a person had 60 INR, they referred to it as having 3 twenty, and for 87 INR they counted it as 4 twenty and 7. Not only this, but the name of week days was not commonly used in this population. They indicate a particular day by reference to whether it occurs before or after the name of the market day of the nearby village. For example, to refer to Monday, they will say they are going to the doctor's camp on the next day of the Silawad (village) bazaar.

The overall population of this project area was so poor that many families were living on less than a dollar a day. Our team therefore developed a very simple and short open-ended questionnaire to record income through work and livestock, crops and non-mobile property, including house and land, to estimate their economic level, which was classified into four categories: Very poor: live in grass huts, no cattle, and depended on manual labor; Poor: live in grass huts, have few cattle and depended on manual labor; Middle: have brick house, cattle and some land; Upper: good house, land and able to provide work to manual labors.

After completion of the survey the data were tabulated and a list of identified cases was prepared. Two professionals in intellectual disability (one is first author of this paper) evaluated all cases on two standard tests; that is, the Developmental Screening Test (DST), and the Vineland Social Maturity Scale (VSMS), adapted for India by Malin and revised by Bharatraj (1992) (22). DST measures development and provides a development quotient (DQ). The VSMS measures social maturity and provides a Social Quotient (SQ) index. SQ approximately correlated with IQ on the Stanford Binet Intelligence Test (BKT) (23). Researchers preferred to take an average of these two test scores (DQ and SQ).

ID professionals on the CBR team preferred these tests because they can be administered in non-clinical settings. Professionals visited the houses of clients for the evaluation, but some cases were also evaluated at the AGT center and in psychiatric camps where the children were brought by their parents. In interventional phases of the program all identified cases were administered two or more IQ tests as per the need and suitability of the test for intervention planning, and to help clients obtain a disability certificate.

The total study population (N=63,789) comprised 24,681 tribal members and 39,108 nontribal participants. The overall prevalence of ID is calculated on the total population (63,789). ID category-wise prevalence is calculated for the total population and separated by gender and tribal/nontribal. Prevalence is defined as the number of cases per 1000 population. The following formula is used to calculate prevalence:

$$\text{Prevalence} = \frac{\text{Number of children with ID}}{\text{Population}} \times 1000$$

FINDINGS

Results are presented in two sections. The first section provides data on the prevalence of ID and the socio-demographic factors associated with it prevalence of ID, which is presented separately for the Tribal and Non-tribal population. In this section, the prevalence of ID is calculated and presented on the combined population, Tribal and Non-Tribal.

Section 1: Socio-demographic profile and prevalence of ID children in Tribal and Non-Tribal Population. Of the children with ID, 202 (77%) lived in poverty. The parents of 200 (76.3%) children had no education. No gender differences were seen in either population (see Table 1). In both population groups (Tribal and non-tribal), males have higher prevalence of ID than females. The overall prevalence of ID in the tribal population is 5.67 per 1,000 (95% CI: 4.24, 7.10), with moderate ID at 2.31 per 1,000, followed by mild and severe categories with the highest prevalence in the Tribal population. The prevalence of ID in the non-tribal population was lower, at 3.11 per 1,000 (95% CI: 2.03, 4.19) population. Similar to the tribal population, the non-tribal population has the same pattern of prevalence in the moderate, mild, and severe categories. The prevalence of profound ID is higher than the borderline category in the tribal population, while the non-tribal population has this in reverse (see Table 2). Calculation of the Odds Ratio (OR = 1.83, CI 95% 1.42 – 2.32) shows that the tribal population has a significantly higher odd of ID than the non-tribal population.

Table 1. Demographics of ID children, gender, poverty level and parental education (n & %)

Characteristics	Subgroups	Number (%)		
		Tribal	Non-Tribal	Total
Gender	Male	73 (27.9)	65 (25.9)	138 (52.7)
	Female	67 (25.6)	57 (21.7)	124 (47.3)
Poverty level	Very poor	78 (29.7)	19 (7.2)	97 (37.0)
	Poor	55 (20.9)	50 (19.0)	105 (40.1)
	Middle	7 (2.6)	47 (17.9)	54 (20.6)
	Upper	0 (0.0)	6 (2.3)	6 (2.3)
Parental Education*	None	139 (53.0)	61 (23.3)	200 (76.3)
	Primary	1 (0.3)	16 (6.1)	17 (6.5)
	Middle	0 (0.0)	21 (8.0)	21 (8.0)
	High school	0 (0.0)	10 (3.8)	10 (3.8)
	Bachelor	0 (0.0)	14 (5.3)	14 (5.3)

* Father.

Table 2. Prevalence of ID in tribal and non-tribal population with gender and ID level

Characteristics	Subgroups	Prevalence			
		Tribal		Non-Tribal	
		N (%)	Prev. (95% CI)	N (%)	Prev. (95% CI)
Gender	Male		2.95 [1.9, 4.0]		1.67 [.88, 2.46]
	Female		2.71 [1.7, 3.72]		1.45 [.71, 2.19]
	Total		5.67 [4.24, 7.1]		3.11 [2.03, 4.19]
ID Level	Borderline	1 (0.71)	.04 [-.08, .16]	4 (3.2)	.10 [-.10, .30]
	Mild	42 (30)	1.7 [.9, 2.5]	37 (30.3)	.95 [.35, 1.55]
	Moderate	57 (40.7)	2.31 [1.38, 3.24]	43 (35.2)	1.1 [.45, 1.75]
	Severe	35 (25)	1.42 [.69, 2.15]	28 (22.9)	.72 [.20, 1.24]
	Profound	5 (3.5)	.20 [-.08, .48]	10 (8.2)	.26 [-.06, .58]
	Total	140 (53.4)	5.67 [4.24, 7.10]	122 (46.6)	3.11[2.03, 4.19]

Prev. = prevalence, reported as cases per 1000.

Section 2: Prevalence of ID children in the combined population (Tribal and Non-Tribal population). Children were grouped into four interval age-groups (3 to 6, 7 to 10, 11 to 14 and 15 to 18 years) for statistical analysis. Prevalence was not distributed equally among the groups. There is an inverse correlation between age and prevalence (ρ = -0.992, 95% CI - 1.38 -0.603) (see Table 3). In the combined tribal and nontribal population, prevalence in males is 2.16 per 1000, which is slightly higher than the female rate of 1.94 per 1000. In both genders the prevalence in ID categories is distributed in the same pattern. That is, highest in moderate ID, followed by mild, severe, profound and borderline ID (see Table 4). There is no significant difference between males and females in the prevalence of ID (Odds ratio = 1.05, 95% CI: 1.42 – 2.32) (see Table 5).

Table 3. Prevalence of ID in different age groups of combined population

Age (Years)	**N**	***Prev.***	**95% CI**	**rho (ρ)***	**95% of CI**
3 to 6	91 (34.7)	1.42	[.69, 2.15]	-.992	[-1.38, -.60]
7 to 10	79 (30.1)	1.24	[.55, 1.93]		
11 to 14	57 (21.7)	0.89	[.31, 1.47]		
15 to 18	35 (13.6)	0.54	[.09, .99]		

* Pearson correlation coefficient.

Table 4. Prevalence of ID categories: In combined population, separated by gender

ID category	**Male**			**Female**		
	N	Prev.	95% CI	N	Prev.	95% CI
Borderline	2 (1.4)	.03	[-.08, .14]	3 (2.4)	.05	[-.09, .19]
Mild	40 (29)	.63	[.14, 1.12]	39 (31.5)	.61	[.13, 1.09]
Moderate	54 (39.1)	.85	[.28, 1.42]	46 (36.1)	.72	[.20, 1.24]
Severe	32 (23.2)	.50	[.06, .94]	31 (25)	.49	[.06, .92]
Profound	10 (7.2)	.16	[-.09, .41]	5 (4)	.08	[-.1, .26]
Total	138 (52.7)	2.16	[1.26, 3.06]	124 (47.3)	1.94	[1.09, 2.79]

Table 5. Odd ratio (OR): Male vs female and tribal vs non-tribal

Categories		Cumulative Incidence	Odd Radio	95% CI
Gender	Male	.0042 (.42)	1.05	[.82, 1.34]
	Female	.004 (.4)		
Population	Tribal	.0057 (.57)	1.83	[1.42, 2.32]
	Non-Tribal	.0031 (.31)		

DISCUSSION

The overall combined prevalence of ID among tribal and non-tribal groups is 0.41%, which is lower than the rates of mental disability of 2.3% reported by Kumar et al. (24) and 2.5% by Srinath and Girimaji (25) in India. Kumar et al. (24) used the Indian Disability Evaluation Assessment Scale (IDEAS) in a cross-sectional door-to-door survey in four randomly selected villages in the state of Karnataka (24). This population has a high literacy rate (94.1%) and higher economic levels compared to our study population. IDEAS is now a government-approved scale for identifying and measuring mental disability since 2002. However, it is not an exclusive indicator of ID as it measures mental disability which originates due to severe mental illness and loss of personal and social skills. Srinath and Girimaji (25) observed a 2% prevalence rate for mild ID (IQ>50) and 0.5% rate for severe (IQ<50) among children who attended child guidance clinics, which is higher than the prevalence we observed in the mixed community (25). In an epidemiologic study conducted in Bangalore of urban and rural children, the Indian Council of Medical Research found a higher overall rate of ID among children < 3 years of age: 1.4% (mild 0.8%, moderate 0.4% and severe 0.2%). This study used ICD-10 criteria for diagnosing ID. The VSMS was used to obtain the Social Quotient, which is approximately equal to IQ (26). This study found a higher prevalence of ID in tribal population (5.67/1,000) than the non-tribal (3.11/1,000). In the literature review, no study was found to compare with these findings.

In the combined tribal and non-tribal population, the prevalence among males is a little higher (2.16/1,000) than among females (1.94/1,000), although this difference is not statistically significant. Other researchers have found a positive correlation between male gender and rural setting with ID prevalence in India (24, 25, 27). Almost three decades ago, low socio-economic status (SES) males had a higher prevalence of ID (7.4/1,000) than females (6.6/1,000) (Nandi et al., 1975 (28). Subsequent decades have witnessed a similar trend. A study conducted two decades ago found a prevalence rate for males of 4.7/1,000 and 1.7/1,000 for females (29). This epidemiological survey was done in 50% of households of 11 villages that were physically very close to the city of Madras, in the state of Tamilnadu, and well connected by road. Parental interviews were conducted and cases were assessed by psychiatrists on ICD-10 criteria of ID (29). This higher ratio of males to females among people with ID is further supported by other researchers in India (25, 27).

We found a higher prevalence of ID (1.42/1,000) in the lower age group of 3 to 6 years, but prevalence reduces as age increases. The group aged 15-18 years had the lowest prevalence rate of ID of 0.54/1,000 (see table 3); indeed, prevalence rates decline as age increases in the combined population. Pearson correlation (ρ - 0.992; 95% CI: -1.38, 0.603) demonstrate an inverse correlation with age and prevalence of ID. A similar propensity of lower prevalence of ID in older compared to younger children is seen in Australia (30). Although this is an important research concern -- why ID prevalence is lower in older children -- the life span of persons with ID is expected equal that of age-matched peers with the advancements in science and technology. However, it is evident in research that the ID population still has a lower life span compared to the non-ID population due, e.g., to high morbidity, chronic diseases and chromosomal disorders (31, 32).

The combined prevalence of moderate, severe and profound ID among both tribal and non-tribal groups (IQ < 49) is 2.79/1,000, and for mild and borderline (IQ > 50), is 1.31/1,000. The prevalence in poor and very poor groups together is 3.17/1,000 and for middle and upper income groups together it is 0.94/1,000. This indicates that ID prevalence is higher in poorer people. The prevalence of more severe disability (IQ < 49) is 1.99/1,000 in middle and upper groups together, which also appears to be lower than among the very poor and poor groups combined (2.12/1,000). Thus, population groups living in poverty have a higher risk of ID. The Odd Ratio of 1.83 demonstrates that the tribal population has a higher risk for ID than the non-tribal population. Possible reasons for this could be poverty, lack of health facilities, genetic disorders, malnutrition, consanguinity, and lack of awareness of treatment facilities. The prevalence of ID is higher (3.14/1,000) among the parents of those with no education than among those who have primary or higher levels of education (0.97/1,000). There is little evidence in the existing scientific literature to confirm the higher prevalence of ID in tribal population in India, except the study conducted by Mehta et al. (1985 (29); that is the closest match, which found a higher rate of mental disability (intellectual disability and severe mental disorders) in schedule caste 15.2/1000 vs. non-scheduled caste 14.1/1000. Most tribal populations are categorized under the schedule casts in India; thus, we assume that this population was tribal.

Strengths and weaknesses

We found a higher prevalence of ID in economically poor populations and more so in the tribal population. This association suggests the value of carrying out further cross-sectional studies in other tribal groups in other states of the country. Persons with ID identified in the survey were found to be true cases when evaluated clinically by professionals. The fact that persons with ID can be identified by less well-educated CBRWs with training in the survey methods and tools used in this study suggests that the cost of data collection can be greatly reduced. However, cases identified on that scale cannot be classified in terms of severity. This could be the first epidemiological study ever conducted on the prevalence of ID in Madhya Pradesh state on both tribal and non-tribal populations.

Conclusion

The prevalence of ID was higher in tribal than in non-tribal populations and also higher among poorer populations. Prevalence is also higher among those whose parents have no education than in those with education up to the primary level or above. The most significant result is that the prevalence of ID declines in both populations with increasing age. A prospective cohort or case-control study can be suggested to determine the reasons behind this tendency. It is a large sample size (N = 63,789), its findings can be generalized for the similar population in Madhya Pradesh. No differences were seen in terms of gender.

Acknowledgments

The first author thanks the Ashagram Trust for the opportunity to conduct this research and to Action Aid for their financial support. He also thanks the CBR team, Dr. Sudipto Chatterjee for allowing him enough freedom to choose instruments and adapt survey methodology. He sincerely thanks to children with ID and their family members, Mr. Prem Ranjan (Action Aid, program officer) for his constant support. The authors did not receive any financial support to write this paper.

References

[1] Maulik PK, Harbour CK. Epidemiology of intellectual disability. In: Stone JH, Blouin M, eds. International encyclopedia of rehabilitation. Buffalo, NY: Center International Rehabilitation Research Information Exchange, 2010. URL: http://cirrie.buffalo.edu/encyclopedia/en/article/144/.

[2] Robertson J, Hatton C, Emerson E, Yasmy MT. The identification of children with, or at significant risk of, intellectual disabilities in low-and middle-income countries: A review. J Appl Res Intellect Disabil 2012;25:99-118.

[3] Chavan BS, Rozatkar AS. Intellectual disability in India: Charity to right based. Indian J Psychiatry 2014;56:113-6.

[4] Durkin M. The epidemiology of developmental disabilities in low-income countries. Ment Retard Dev Disabil Res Rev 2002;8:206-11.

[5] National Sample Survey Organisation. Disabled persons in India. NSS 58th round (July- December 2002). New Delhi: Ministry Statistics Programme Implementation, Government of India, 2002.

[6] Statistical Profile of Scheduled Tribes in India. New Delhi: Ministry Tribal Affairs Statistics Division, Government of India, 2013. URL: http://tribal.nic.in/WriteRead Data/userfiles/file/Statistics/StatisticalProfileofSTs2013.pdf.

[7] Kate SL. Health problems of tribal population groups from the state of Maharashtra. Indian J Med Sci 2001;55:99-108.

[8] Balgir RS. Tribal health problems, disease burden and ameliorative challenges in tribal communities with special emphasis on tribes of Orissa. Proceedings of National Symposium on Tribal Health 2006:161-76. URL: http://citeseerx.ist.psu. edu/viewdoc/download?doi=10.1.1.515.1245&rep=rep1&type=pdf.

[9] Chatterjee S, Patel V, Chatterjee A, Weiss H. Evaluation of a community-based rehabilitation model for chronic schizophrenia in rural India. Br J Psychiatry 2003;182:57-62.

[10] Mercadante MT, Evans-Lacko S, Paula CS. Perspectives of intellectual disability in Latin American countries: Epidemiology, policy, and services for children and adults. Curr Opin Psychiatry 2009;22:469-74.

[11] Girimaji SC, Srinath S. Perspectives of intellectual disability in India: Epidemiology, policy, services for children and adults. Curr Opin Psychiatry, 23, 441-6.

[12] Narayanan HS. A study of the prevalence of mental retardation in Southern India. Int J Ment Health 1981;10:28-36.

[13] Belmont L. Screening for severe mental retardation in developing countries: The international pilot study of severe childhood disability. In: Berg JM, ed. Science and service in mental retardation. London: Methuen, 1986:389-95.

[14] Kumar GS. Are the disability data in India appropriate? Natl Med J India 2009;22:278.

[15] Lakhan R, Mawson AR. Identifying children with intellectual disabilities in the tribal population of Barwani district in state of Madhya Pradesh, India. J Appl Res Intellect Disabil 2016;29:211-9.

[16] Robertson J, Emerson E, Hatton C, Yasamy MT. Efficacy of community-based rehabilitation for children with or at significant risk of intellectual disabilities in low- and middle-income countries: A review. J Appl Res Intellect Disabil 2012;25:143–54.

[17] Girimaji SC. Clinical practice guidelines for the diagnosis and management of children with mental retardation. Indian J Psychiatry 2008;49:43-67.

[18] Grossman HJ. Classification in mental retardation, revised ed. Washington, DC: American Association Mental Deficiency, 1983.

[19] Census of India, Census Data online. Government of India, Ministry of Home Affairs. URL: http://censusindia.gov.in/2011-common/censusdataonline.html.

[20] Arya S. Screening of pre-school children for early identification of developmental disabilities in rural area. Indian J Clin Psychol 1991;18:65-70.

[21] Madhwan T, Menon DK, Kalyan M, Narayan J, Subbarao TA. Mental retardation. A manual for village rehabilitation workers. Hyderabad: National Institute Mentally Handicapped, 1988.

[22] Bharatraj J. Vineland Social Maturity Scale. Indian adaptation: Enlarged version, Mysore: Swayamsiddha Prakashanam, 1992.

[23] Kishore MT, Nizamie SH, Nizamie A. Utility of Reiss Sscreen in identifying psychiatric problems in persons with mental retardation. Indian J Psychol Med 2010;32:38 -41.

[24] Srinath S, Girimaji SR. Epidemiology of child and adolescent mental health problems and mental retardation. NIMHANS J 1999;17:355-66.

[25] Srinath S, Girimaji SC, Gururaj G, Seshadri S, Subbakrishna DK, Bhola P, et al., Epidemiological study of child and adolescent psychiatric disorders in urban and rural areas of Bangalore, India. Indian J Med Res 2005;122:67-79.

[26] Sharma S, Raina SK, Bhardwaj AK, Chaudhary S, Kashyap V, Chander V. Socio demography of mental retardation: A community-based study from a goitre zone in rural sub-Himalayan India. J Neurosci Rural Pract 2015;6:165-9.

[27] Kumar GS, Das A, Bhandary PV, Soans, SJ, Kumar HHN, Kotian MS. Prevalence and pattern of mental disability using Indian disability evaluation assessment scale in a rural community of Karnataka. Indian J Psychiatry 2008;50:21–3.

[28] Nandi DN, Ajmany S, Ganguli H, Banerjee G, Boral GC, Ghosh A, et al., Psychiatric disorders in a rural community in West Bengal: An epidemiological study. Indian J Psychiatry 1975;17:87-99.

[29] Mehta P, Joseph A, Verghese A. An epidemiological study of psychiatric disorders in a rural area in Tamil Nadu. Indian J Psychiatry 1985;27:153-8.

[30] Leonard H, Petterson B, Bower C, Sanders R. Prevalence of intellectual disability in Western Australia. Pediatr Perinat Epidemiol 2003;17:58-67.

[31] Hosking FJ, Carey IM, Shah SM, Harris T, DeWilde S, Beighton C, et al. Mortality among adults with intellectual disability in England: Comparisons with the general population. Am J Public Health 2016;106:1483-90.

[32] Bear MF, Huber KM, Warren ST. The mGluR theory of fragile X mental retardation. Trends Neurosci 2014;27:370-7.

In: Intellectual Disability
Editors: Ariel Tenenbaum et al.
ISBN: 978-1-53617-866-1

Chapter 4

THE EXPERIENCES OF CARING FOR CHILDREN WITH INTELLECTUAL DISABILITIES: PERSPECTIVES FROM SELECTED SPECIAL SCHOOLS IN ASHANTI REGION OF GHANA

Mprah Wisdom Kwadwo, PhD, MPhil, Acheampong Enoch*, MSc and Bediako Joseph

Centre for Disability and Rehabilitation Studies,
Department of Community Health,
Kwame Nkrumah University of Science and Technology,
Kumasi, Ghana

* Corresponding Author: Enoch Acheampong, Lecturer, Centre for Disability and Rehabilitation Studies, Department of Community Health, Kwame Nkrumah University of Science and Technology, Kumasi, Ghana. E-mail: caposterl@yahoo.com.

ABSTRACT

The relevance of caregiving cannot be overlooked as long as people are getting older, contracting chronic illness, having disabilities and certain protracted ailments. This study sought to explore the challenges facing caregivers of children with intellectual disability in three selected special schools in the Ashanti Region of Ghana. Methods: A qualitative exploratory study was carried out in which simple random and purpose sampling techniques were used. In-depth interview was used to collect data. Data transcription was done using the notes taken during the interview and comparing it with information recorded on audio tapes. Dominant themes were developed and coded through data-led approach and have been presented as the major findings. Results: The study revealed that children with intellectual disability tend to forget what they are taught the previous day. The absence of incentives such as risk and overtime allowance affects house mothers. Conclusion: It is recommended that stakeholders should provide more facilities such as classrooms and dormitories for special schools and revise and improve the conditions of service of staff of special schools.

INTRODUCTION

Intellectual disability (ID) is a condition that significantly decreases one's ability to comprehend, learn and apply different and intricate information or skills, affecting individual's inability to live independent life. The condition starts before adulthood with a long-term effect on development (1). This definition implies that individuals with intellectual disability suffer a lifetime functional and developmental problems which affect their effective participation in society.

Caregiving is the act and process of attending to the daily needs of another person. The person may be a relative, a spouse, or friend (2). Usually, care recipients have certain conditions and need help in activities of daily living such as bathing, toileting, eating and dressing (3). Quality caregiving that comes from the heart has the ability to promote the physical, emotional, mental, spiritual and social well-being of the care receiver; and it also helps lift and cheer care recipients to have hope and enjoy life (4). Research has proven that quality caregiving promotes the psychological, emotional, physical and social wellbeing of care recipients especially children with ID (5). This include but not limited to activities such as aiding the person with ID to visit a doctor, assisting with personal care, providing support during meal preparation, transportation or supporting the person to do laundry.

Although caregiving is essential in promoting the wellbeing of those in need of assistance, studies have shown that caregivers experience numerous challenges. These challenges are the results child's physical, emotional, and financial demands and include depression, emotional strain, anxiety, boredom, isolation, sleeplessness, helplessness and frustration (6).

This is especially serious for carer of children with emotional and behavioral challengessuch as children with ID. It has been estimated that about 15% and 33% of carers of children with ID have health and emotional problems resulting from assisting children with ID (7).

Some researchers have found that there is a relationship between caring for children with ID and economic burden. Caring for children with ID can result in three levels of economic cost: employment- related (income benefit, employee productivity and forfeiting career opportunities), out of-pocket (expenditures on the person, expenditures on help, money transfers, costs of relocation, and transportation and unpaid care labour (8). What this means is that caregivers of ID children are likely to lose their jobs because they have to spend much time with these children with little or no time to engage in income generation and economic ventures. The most worrying aspect of all these is that caregivers tend to accept these challenges and do not see them as a burden because the challenges become part of them with time (8).

There are limited data on caregiving for children with ID in Ghana, especially challenges facing caregivers. This is due to the fact that little has been done on caregiving in Ghana. The main objective of the study was to ascertain the challenges caregivers of ID children face with special focus on careers from some selected special schools in the Kumasi Metro. Findings provided understanding on the challenges of caregivers of children with ID, which is vital to effective response to their concerns.

OUR STUDY

The study was carried out in three special schools within the Kumasi Metro. The schools are Garden City Special School, Community Special Vocational Training School and Edwinase Rehabilitation Center. These schools provide vocational training and life skills for children with ID.The population for the study included teachers and housemothers who had worked with the schools for at least three years as well as parents of ID children, who are enrolled in the three selected schools. A total of thirty participants made up of 12 teachers, nine parents and nine housemothers took part in the study. The housemothers are employed by the school to assist the children in their daily life activities.

The researchers used both random and purposive sampling techniques to select the participants. Purposive sampling was used to select teachers and housemothers who could provide adequate information on the challenges they encountered caring for children with ID while simple random sampling was used to select the parents. A qualitative study, using face-to-face in-depth interview, was conducted to collect data from participants. An interview guide with open-questions was used to collect the data. The interview was tape recorded with audio tape recorder.

The audio recordings from the three categories of participants were transcribed differently and verbatim by the researchers. Transcripts were coded to identify the dominant themes based on the research questions. Coding was undertaken by a team of three research assistants under the supervision of the researchers. The emerging themes from the data were analysed in duplicate, with each analyst blind to the summary of the other. After developing the themes, the two analysts compared their respective summaries, reconciled difference, and then merged the major themes. Extra readers were invited to help resolve any differences between summaries from the two analysts. Direct quotations of some of the responses were used to support the themes.

Ethical consideration

Ethical approval was obtained from the Committee on Human Research, Publications and Ethics, Kwame Nkrumah University of Science and Technology, School of Medical Sciences and Komfo Anokye Teaching Hospital. As with the principle of voluntarism, participants were told participation in the study was voluntary and were free to withdraw from the study at any time. They were assured of their confidentiality and anonymity through the removal of all identifiers from the research instrument.

FINDINGS

The majority of the participants were below the age of 50 years, and more females than males took part in the study, probably because all the caretakers (housemothers) were females, and also, all the parents who were available for selection were females. In terms of education, half of the participants had tertiary education (the teachers and parents) while few were middle school leavers (house mothers) (see Table 1).

Challenges

The study revealed that caregivers who took part in the study faced several challenges; however the different categories of caregivers faced different challenges. The findings are therefore been presented under the following headings; challenges facing parents, house mothers and teachers.

The challenges parents encountered ranged from issues relating to appreciation of their children's condition, through physical and psychological problems, to financial difficulties.

Table 1. Demographic characteristics of the respondents

Variables	Frequency (N=30)	Percentage (%)
Status of caregivers		
Head Teachers	3	10
Teachers	9	30
House mothers	9	30
Parents	9	30
Total	30	100
Gender		
Males	9	30
Females	21	70
Total	30	100
Age group		
30-39 years	11	37
40-49 years	10	33
50-59 years	9	30
Total	30	100
Educational status	9	
Middle School Leavers	6	30
Senior High School	15	20
Tertiary	30	50
Total		100

The study found that the major challenge facing parents related to appreciating their child's condition. Most of the parents asserted that the sadness and guilt accumulating in their hearts had not varnished completely and that they could not understand why their wards had the impairment. One parent said that "When I compare my son over here with his other siblings at home, in fact, it is not easy for me to believe that he is my son" while another said: "I simply do not believe why I have given birth to such a child. Sometimes, I wonder what the actual problem is as far as the condition of my child is concerned."

Another related challenge the parents mentioned is the physical and psychological impact of caring for children with ID. The psychological burden revealed by the parents included sadness, thinking and worrying, stress, and the fear of who would care for their wards after their death. One parent remarked: "I fear for my daughter because I don't think people will love and care for her the way I do, after my death."

It was also revealed that for parents of children who required frequent assistance, the psychological issues were compounded by the stress of providing everyday care and the taunts from neighbours and community members. Another parent also said: "Rarely do I walk with my daughter… because people will be looking at us in the streets and I feel uncomfortable because people kept staring at us."

Financial burden

Again, the study found that the parents had difficulties in raising funds to support the cost of taking care of their children who have ID. Most of the parents said the cost involved in taking care of a child with ID is higher than the cost of caring for a child without ID. For example, a parent said that "I have to take my son to hospital for check-up almost every month and this is putting a lot of financial difficulties on me especially because I am a single mother."

However, a few of the parents whose wards had no additional disabilities asserted that, there was no significant difference between the cost of taking care of a child with disability and those without disability.

Obtaining Admission for Their Wards

Responses from the participants revealed that getting admission in the special schools for their wards was a major challenge for most of the parents. Most of the parents indicated that they had to wait for several years before they could secure admission for their wards. This puts a lot of pressure on the parents, and also, impacted negatively on their economic situation since they sometimes had to miss work in order to attend to the needs of their children. One of the parents commented: "In fact the number of special schools in the Ashanti Region is few. And one of the problems we face is securing admission for our wards.....The schools do not have enough buildings to accommodate the students." Another parent supported this assertion:

> "This is not the first school I came to look for admission for my child. I was unable to secure admission in the special school that was close to me [and] that is why I brought my son here......and even here, I was made to wait for six months before I was finally given the green light to bring him here."

Experiences of House Mothers as caregivers

The findings indicated that house mothers in the three special schools encountered several challenges: exposure to infections, mobilizing the pupils and low remuneration.

Most of the house mothers indicated their continuous contact with the children exposed them to diseases such as flue and skin rashes.

> Sometimes we get infected with catarrh, flue and skin disease. We are always becoming sick due to our contact with the students...most of these students are always sick and in our attempt to attend to their needs, end up contracting those ailments. They are overcrowded in their rooms so they easily fall sick and the sickness spread quickly to others of which we are no exception. (Housemother 2)

However, some of the house mothers disputed the above claim and mentioned they were never exposed to such risks and that even if they did, they could not attribute it to their contact with the children.

Mobilizing the pupils

According to the mothers, they often had difficulties to mobilizing the children to perform their daily tasks such as getting them to the dining hall to eat due to the children's behavior challenges.

> "Some of the pupils are very difficult to attend to. They become restless most of the time and you gather some at one place and if you decide to leave them in order to get other, by the time you come back they have all scattered and you have to bring them back one after the other. This makes it difficult to get them together and also makes our work difficult." (Housemother 3)

Some also said they often got frustrated and stressed up due the pressure on them to hurriedly dress up the children for classes.

> "Because of the high pupil-house mother ratio, sometimes class hours may be due but the students may not be ready. This often led to a state of confusion, frustration, stress and frequent headaches." (Housemother 1)

Poor working conditions

It was also found that in spite of the nature of their work, the house mothers are not paid well and did not received overtime and risk allowances. They also indicated that there was no opportunity to be promoted.

> "Our salary is very small, but there is nothing I can do. I don't have money to start a business of my own so I am managing it" Also, I have not been promoted before even though I have worked with the school for the past ten years." (Housemother 5)

Challenges confronting teachers as caregivers

One major challenge confronting the teachers in all the selected schools was the issue of pupils' inability to understand what they were taught. All the teachers asserted that the process of acquiring various skills such as self-help skills, life skills, gross motor skills, self-care skills and fine motor skill was slow because of the relatively low Intelligent Quotient and attention span of the pupils. They lamented that they always taught the concepts which was a bit stressful.

> "You teach them today and by tomorrow they have forgotten everything that they were taught the previous day."

> "Teaching these children is very monotonic because one self-help skills and life skills have to be taught over and over for long time because they always forget what they we teach them.

Another challenge confronting the teachers is overcrowding in the class rooms due to inadequate facilities to accommodate the children.

> "The class size is too large considering the conditions of these children….this has affected the quality of activities we carry out as teachers." (Teacher 2)

DISCUSSION

The study has revealed that carers of children with intellectual disabilities experience several challenges. The challenges vary depending on the role the individual carer performed. For parents, the challenges were associated with physical and psychological problems, difficulty in obtaining admission for their children as well as difficulty in appreciating their children's conditions while housemothers' challenges were concerned with exposure to infections, poor working conditions and difficulty in mobilizing the children. The teachers also complained of repetitive and routine teaching as a result of ID children's inability to understand what they are taught as well as large class sizes.

The challenges encountered by caregivers in performing their duties are expected and consistent with previous studies. Previous studies have shown that caring is associated with a lot of complications such as severe depression, emotional strain, anxiety, boredom, isolation, sleeplessness, low morale, helplessness feeling, and frustration (7).

These challenges may be worse if caregivers lack support services and training to handle the behavior problems of the children. caregivers of children with ID are unable to understand and appreciate their conditions if they lack basic skills and training (8). Parents, in particular, are likely to encounter numerous challenges because they play different roles in the life of children with ID. These roles include caring for them, providing their physical needs, and also helping them to carry out simple activities of daily living. It is also reported that most parents of children with ID especially those in developing countries usually find it difficult to appreciate their wards' condition due to lack of access to information about disability (9).

On the part of teachers, it was found that the major challenge confronting them was the class size. They complained that there are large class size which affects quality teaching and learning. This condition does not permit the teachers to have enough time to attend to the varying learning needs of the children. In view of this finding, the conclusion that the teaching and learning process for children with ID requires patience and love holds true.

Limitation of the study

The major limitation of the study was that it focused on only special schools in the Kumasi metro, with a very limited sample size. Although there will be the temptation to generalize the findings, any such interpretation should done with caution.

CONCLUSION

The challenges facing the parents were: financial burden, difficulty in securing admission for their children, understanding and appreciating the condition of their children as well as physical and psychological health impact. The house mothers are also confronted with the following challenges: Susceptibility to infectious and other communicable diseases, difficulty in mobilizing the children to carry out specific activities and lack of incentives such as promotion risk or overtime allowance. On the part of the teachers, the study found that the major challenge confronting them is the repetitive nature of their work due to the fact that the children always forget what they are taught as well as large class size which affects effective teaching and classroom work.

Implications of the study

Based on the research findings, the following recommendations have been made. It is recommended that parents with children with intellectual disability should form self-help groups where they can meet to share ideas. This will go a long way in helping them deal with the psychological and emotional problems they go through due to the condition of their children. This is because caregivers of children with ID who lack basic skills, training and support services are unable to understand and appreciate their children's conditions.

In addition, it is recommended that administrators of Ghana Education Trust Fund (GETFUND) should provide more facilities such as classrooms and dormitories for special schools in order to avoid overcrowding and its associated health effects.

Again, it is recommended that the Government of Ghana, through the Finance and Employment Ministries, should revise the conditions of service of special education teachers and house mothers to provide them with risk allowance, overtime allowance and responsibility allowance.

Finally, it is recommended that further studies should be done on the role of caregivers and support systems available to caregivers of children with intellectual disabilities in Ghana.

ACKNOWLEDGMENTS

Authors did not receive any external financial support. We wish to thank the authorities of the various special schools who allowed us to conduct the study in their schools.

REFERENCES

[1] World Health Organisation. Mental health definition: Intellectual disability. URL: www.euro.who.int/.../health...health/.../definition-intellectual-disability.

[2] National Alliance for Caregiving. Caregiving in the United States, 2004. URL: www.caregiving.org/data/04finalreport.pdf.

[3] Green R, Barth RP, Webb MB, Wall A, Gibbons C, Craig C. Characteristics of out-of home caregiving environments provided under child welfare services. Child Welfare 2008;87(3):5.

[4] Le J. Essence of caregiver: The Importance of caregiving, 2011. URL: essenceofcaregiver.blogspot.com/2011/07/importance-of-care-giving.html.

[5] Guberman N. Caregivers: Their role in rehabilitation. Buffalo, NY: Center International Rehabilitation Research Information Exchange (CIRRIE), 2010.

[6] Brody EM. Prospects for family caregiving. In: Kane RA, Penrod JD, eds. Family caregiving in an aging society. Thousand Oaks, CA: Sage, 1995:15-28.

[7] Desforges C. The impact of parental involvement, parental support and family education on pupil achievement and adjustment: A review of literature. London: DfES Publications, 2003.

[8] Young HM, Zhang J, Vitaliano PP. Is caregiving a risk factor for illness? Curr Direct Psychol Sci 2004;13(1):13-6.

[9] World Health Organisation. Supporting informal caregivers of people living with dementia, 2012. URL: www.who.int/mental_health/neurology/.../dementia_thematicbrief_informal_care.pdf.

In: Intellectual Disability
Editors: Ariel Tenenbaum et al.
ISBN: 978-1-53617-866-1

Chapter 5

The Quality of Life of Normally Achieving and Low-Achieving Participants: Is It Associated with IQ and Metacognition?

Yasser A Al-Hilawani*
Department of Counseling and Educational Psychology,
Faculty of Education, Yarmouk University, Irbid, Jordan

Abstract

In this chapter, I tested the notion that performances on the IQ test, the Mooney problem checklist as a reflection of the quality of life (QoL), and metacognition were intercorrelated. It was also intended to find if there were significant differences between the normally achieving and the low-achieving participants on the Mooney scale and on the metacognitive instrument (i.e., the metacognitive test, reaction time, and the metacognitive test scores divided by mean reaction time) when

* Corresponding Author: Professor Yasser A Al-Hilawani, EdD, Department of Counseling and Educational Psychology, Faculty of Education, Yarmouk University, Irbid, Jordan. Email: yhilawani@netscape.net.

controlling for the effect of influencing variables. Results revealed that only the performance of the normally achieving participants was consistent with the notion stated. The heterogeneity of the low-achieving group was presented as one of the many explanations for the lack of significant association between their performances on the three measures. Overall, participants with high IQs obtained high scores on the metacognitive test; and older participants obtained better scores on the metacognitive test and on the metacognitive test scores divided by mean reaction time compared to younger ones. The analysis showed no significant differences existed between the two participating groups in responding to items on the Mooney scale or the metacognitive instrument when controlling for influencing variables. Insights, discussions, and suggestions for future research were presented.

INTRODUCTION

This study was conducted to test the hypothesis that intelligent quotient (i.e., IQ scores), performance on the Mooney problem checklist as a reflection of the quality of life (QoL), and individuals' metacognitive performances in real-life situations were intercorrelated. This hypothesis, if confirmed, would reveal if QoL could be significantly affected by IQ and by metacognition when using normally achieving and low-achieving participants. It was derived from recent research with hearing and deaf and hard-of-hearing (D/HH) volunteers which showed that performances on these three measures were significantly correlated with each other (1). This current study also tested the hypothesis that no significant differences would be found in metacognition and responses on the Mooney scale between the normally achieving and low-achieving participants when controlling for the effect of influencing variables (e.g., IQ). The term low-achievement referred, in this study, to a heterogeneous group of participants labeled officially slow learners by the Ministry of Education in the State of Kuwait. As described later in the study, this group included all individuals with mild disabilities as well as misdiagnosed students all of whom enrolled in a special education program implemented within the regular school setting.

Historically, the QoL concept had been approached in special education in the early days when contemplating euthanasia (i.e., mercy killing) to decide whether the individuals with severe disabilities ought to live (2, 3). They were regarded at that time as a burden that jeopardized the prosperity and the future of society, especially in the case of economic strait, where institutionalizations, for example, put more constraints on society (4). Early efforts to assist individuals with disabilities were restricted to persons with mild intellectual disabilities to prepare them to return to society and to live independently as much as possible (5).

The basic connotation in the QoL concept, when applied to individuals with disabilities in early days, was whether or not they were considered autonomous and self-determining members of the society (2); and the possibility that they would be enjoying life in the future regardless of their disabling conditions or the inability of the society to accommodate their needs. When considering that a person would not have a QoL, this person was then not worth living and vice versa (6). The QoL domains included at that time were the severity of the disability, the prediction for future development and suffering, and the stress and demands of persons with disabilities put on the family and the services available in the community (7).

The perception of QoL has been evolving since then due to civility and to the introduction of laws and legislation such as the Individuals with Disabilities Education Improvement Act-IDEA (8). The antiquated notion that individuals with severe disabilities were not people or "nonpersons" who lacked the capacity for meaningful interaction with others has changed. The concept of life started to be viewed as an irreducible entity and of equal value for all people with and without disabilities (9). This shift in thinking and practice led to pursue better QoL for all individuals including persons with disabilities. Viewing individuals as different in characteristics but not in essence paved the way to the inclusion movement to educate individuals with disabilities alongside their non-disabled peers.

One view to QoL is to consider it "as individuals' perception of their position in life in the context of the culture and value systems in which they live and in relation to their goals, expectations, standards and concerns" (10). Based on this definition, QoL relates to various aspects of the individuals' lives; and it is influenced by the physical and psychological conditions, the degree of independence, social relationships, and the personal ways of life and their relationship to relevant features in the surrounding environment. According to this view, QoL is regarded as multidimensional and predisposed to personal and environmental factors (11, 12). It is also subjective feelings related to one's own well-being and life satisfaction which should be examined within a cultural context to determine what elements constitute QoL (13). This indicates that QoL as a complex construct is not constant; it is evolving over time within and across cultures with varying degrees of emphasis.

In sum, QoL impacts the lives of all people. Suggested domains to QoL have been proposed by the World Health Organization (10, 12, 13). These domains have been reflected in another set of domains introduced by Verdugo et al. (14); they were interpersonal relations, social inclusion, personal development, physical well-being, self-determination, material well-being, emotional well-being, family, recreation and leisure, safety/security, and environment (home/residence/living situation). Verdugo and colleagues (14) suggested principles and guidelines that should assist in the measurement of QoL which include valued life experiences as seen by the individual; the introduced domains contributing to interconnected and full life experiences; the physical, social, and cultural conditions seen important to individuals; and addressing and evaluating experiences common to people as well as to individuals.

While QoL has been studied in the west for many years among groups with severe disabilities (3, 7, 15), it has not been explored among individuals identified as low-achieving students and labeled as slow learners especially in the State of Kuwait. This is the case due to the relatively short history of the field of special education not only in Kuwait but also other surrounding countries (16). Searching the literature did not reveal such studies using low-achieving individuals in Kuwait or in other Arab countries such as Oman, Qatar, Bahrain, Saudi Arabia, and Jordan. Due to the lack of appropriate and adequate diagnostic tools, this group might be formed of borderline functioning individuals; individuals with learning, mild intellectual, or emotional disabilities; and/ or underachievers/low-achievers. Personnel working in the field of special education and the available diagnostic tools could not validly and reliably differentiate individuals who have learning problems due to environmental factors from individuals who have intrinsic learning disabilities or others classified under the term mild disabilities (16).

Bearing in mind that low-achievement is not a proper classification in special education and that individuals in this group are heterogeneous, will they differ in QoL as measured by the Mooney scale when compared with normally achieving participants? Is performance on the Mooney scale associated with IQ and with metacognition?

Literature showed that IQ influences various facets of life like an educational achievement, employment prospects and wealth generation, career outcome, and well-being (17). Nota et al. (18) stated that participants with severe intellectual disabilities exhibited the lowest levels of QoL, social abilities, and self-determination (e.g., making decisions, expressing opinions, thoughts, or emotions). The authors reported that the IQ score and the basic social skills predicted membership in the high or low QoL groups; that IQ contributed significantly to positive QoL and self-determination; that self-determination and QoL were significantly correlated; and that one's social abilities assumed an important role in learning, in coping with daily life events, in establishing and maintaining interaction with others, and in achieving a satisfactory degree of social acceptance and better QoL.

When it comes to metacognition (19, 20) in special education, one orientation is to consider it as an alternative approach to measuring cognitive development. It has been advanced as analyzing simultaneously, in a visual-spatial perception manner, common and distinctive features of daily life experiences to construct knowledge and to reach an understanding of one's surroundings (21). Metacognition is regarded, in this sense, a feature of intelligent ability that involves activation, cultivation, and mobilization of one's higher-order thinking processes for effective functioning in life (22). Al-Hilawani and Abdullah (23) showed significant correlations between IQ scores, metacognitive test scores, total reaction time, and metacognitive test scores divided by time in the low-achievement group labeled slow learners. The authors mentioned that intelligence plays a significant role in the correlation between achievement and metacognition and that the concept of metacognition is related to the concept of intelligence (24, 25). In an earlier study, Al-Hilawani et al. (26) revealed significant differences in metacognition among students with normal hearing, D/HH, low-achieving, and institutionally raised students. Al-Hilawani et al. (26) showed that the D/HH and normally hearing students performed significantly higher than the low-achieving students and the students institutionally raised. The low-achieving and institutionally raised students did not show significant differences in the test of metacognition and in the test scores divided by time.

The QoL issue may be related to IQ, to metacognition as measured in real-life situations, and to social and behavioral status because all of them are linked to how individuals function and succeed in their environments (1). This present study was conducted to examine the relationship between these variables when administered to two groups of participants, the normally achieving and low-achieving males and females from the State of Kuwait. The second aim was to find whether or not there were significant differences between the two groups of participants on the above measures. The independent variables were normally achieving and low-achieving males and females. The dependent variables were the performances on the metacognitive test, the metacognitive test scores divided by time, reaction time, and responses on the Mooney scale. The research questions were:

- Is there a significant correlation between performances on the metacognitive instrument (i.e., metacognitive test, reaction time, and metacognitive test scores divided by time) and the Mooney scale, on the one hand, and the students' age and IQ score, on the other hand?
- Is there a significant difference between the two groups of participants on the Mooney scale when controlling for the effect of influencing variables (e.g., IQ)?

- Is there a significant difference between the two groups of participants on the metacognitive instrument when controlling for the effect of influencing variables (e.g., IQ)?

It was hypothesized that significant relationships would exist between the measures used; and that no significant differences would exist between the two groups of participants on these measures when controlling for significantly contributing variables. Previous research (1) revealed significant negative correlations between scores on the Mooncy scale, on the one hand, and reaction time and IQ scores, on the other hand, meaning that a high score on the Mooney was associated with a less reaction time on the metacognitive measure and with a low score on the IQ test; and participants with high IQs obtained high scores on the metacognitive test. Al-Hilawani concluded that the social and adjustment problems could not be addressed in isolation from significantly contributing factors such as the IQ for the hearing and D/HH individuals; that school achievement affected QoL as measured by the Mooney scale; and that the IQ was the link between performances on the Mooney scale and the metacognitive measure.

MY STUDY

Two groups totaling eighty-eight participants volunteered for this study by the means of initial personal contact with their teachers. Data collection started after meeting all the ethical guidelines for obtaining all the required agreements. The teachers in participating schools assisted in obtaining the necessary consents. The first group consisted of 42 normally achieving males and females (mean age = 17.10 years, SD = 1.07 years, age range = 15.45 to 19.10 years). There were 21 males (mean age = 16.41 years, SD = .97 years, age range = 15.45 to 18.70 years) and 21 females (mean age = 17.79 years, SD = .61 years, age range = 16.12 to 19.10). Participants in this group had no history of academic difficulties; they were not previously retained at any school grade level.

The second group consisted of 46 low-achieving males and females (mean age = 16.07 years, SD = 1.42 years, age range = 14.19 to 20.08 years). There were 25 males (mean age = 16.06 years, SD = 1.59 years, age range = 14.39 to 20.08 years) and 21 females (mean age = 16.09 years, SD = 1.24 years, age range = 14.19 to 19.58 years). The IQ scores of participants in this group ranged roughly from 70 to 85. They were taught in separate classrooms with a class load of 10 students; they were labeled officially slow learners by the Ministry of Education. They received academic instructions in self-contained special education classrooms located within the regular school buildings. Participants in this group obtained failing grades, studied a modified version of the regular curriculum, and some of them were retained previously. As stated in the literature (e.g., 27), this group is heterogeneous and formed of students who have not been receiving proper academic instructions; or they are borderline low functioning students; or students with mild intellectual, learning, or emotional disabilities. Therefore, the low-achievement term is a description of this heterogeneous group and a reflection of the lack of valid and reliable assessment tools along with inadequate preparation of educational diagnosticians (see 16) for details on this topic and for guidelines concerning identifying students with suspected learning disabilities who fall under the umbrella of low-achievement or underachievement).

Instrumentation

Three instruments were used to collect the data for this study. The first one was the Raven Standard Progressive Matrices Scale (28). This test targets capabilities such as abstract and analytical thinking, visual-spatial perception, and cognitive flexibility. According to the testing manual, this test has a reliability coefficient (alpha) rating between .81 to .91.

The second instrument was The Mooney Problem Checklist (29). This instrument was used as an indication of QoL since its areas mentioned below were reflected in the tool developed by the World Health

Organization - WHO (30). The WHO tool covers domains like physical, psychological, level of independence, social relationships, environment, and spirituality/religion/personal beliefs. The Mooney scale was applied in this current study because the items selected were applicable to participants and could be used at a personal level. Also, the WHO instrument does not limit or exclude questions or items as related to QoL if they are culturally relevant and/or applicable to individuals with special needs like the case with inclusion, empowerment, self-determination, and general well-being. Responses to these areas, or domains, or items were considered self-reported perceptions. They were modified in the Mooney instrument from its original form (i.e., underlining all items that reflected participants' areas of concern while circling the ones of greatest concern to them) to a four-point Likert-type scale format. The Likert format was considered suitable for this study because many of the stated problems existed among people at various degrees of intensity (1).

One hundred fifty four items were selected for this study. The selected items were judged suitable and applicable to the local culture as viewed by five different reviewers working in the field of education. These items were first translated from English to Arabic by a translator and then back-translated by a second translator to reveal content and meaning discrepancy. All items were read aloud to all participants to control for reading difficulty. Participants were asked to respond to each stated problem by selecting the choice not applicable (assigned 1 point), rarely (assigned 2 points), sometimes (assigned 3 points), or always (assigned 4 points). A higher score on this tool would indicate more problems and less satisfaction; a lower score would indicate otherwise. One hundred fifty one items correlated positively with the total score. The non-significant positive items (n=11) ranged in correlation from (.01) to (.19.). The non-significant negative items (n=3) ranged in correlation from (-.01) to (-.05). The overall reliability coefficient (alpha) after removing all non-significant items (i.e., 14 items) was .95. The final 140 selected items, with significant positive correlations, ranged from (.20) to (.48), covered the following 11 areas:

1) Health and Physical Development (HPD – Items = 7).
2) Finance, Living Condition, and Employment (FLE - Items = 7).
3) Social and Recreational Activities (SRA - Items = 12).
4) Social-Psychological Relations (SPR – Items = 22).
5) Personal-Psychological Relations (PPR – Items = 17).
6) Courtship, Sex, and Marriage (CSM – Items =14).
7) Morals and Religion (MR – Items = 13).
8) Adjustment to School Work (ASW – Items = 13).
9) Home and Family (HF – Items = 14).
10) Curriculum and Teaching Procedure (CTP – Items = 14).
11) The Future: Vocational and Educational (FVE – Items = 7).

The subtotal of each of the 11 areas of the Mooney checklist was computed by adding up relevant items and then dividing the outcome by the number of items in that area.

The third tool was the metacognitive instrument (26). The content of this instrument was drawn from naïve psychology, naïve physics, and naïve biology domains (31). Examples of naïve psychology covered psychological states such as desire, sadness, happiness, anger, fear, disgust, surprise, and pain. These states were primarily portrayed by facial expressions, unlike the contents of the physics and biology domains. Examples of naïve biology included identifying and understanding the processes of reproduction, classification, inheritance, illness, organic growth, death, and eating and sleeping. Examples of naïve physics included presenting pictures to determine cause-effect relationships, identifying, classifying, and understanding physical objects transformations.

The metacognitive instrument was formed of 54 items. These items represented the three knowledge domains in the following manner: 19 items representing the psychology domain (8 items depicting situations with real people while 11 items using cartoon drawings), 17 items representing the physics domain (15 items were cartoon drawings while 2 items were real pictures), and 18 items representing the biology domain in cartoon drawings (1).

Initially, this instrument was reviewed and evaluated by five faculty members in the College of Education to decide if its items targeted participants' reasoning and problem-solving skills using the knowledge of real-life problems and situations. Reviewers examined the accuracy and the relationship between each target picture and the four choices and whether the target picture matched with or related appropriately to the correct option. Reviewers' suggestions and recommendations were all implemented.

The 54 test items were then put in an electronic format to add in the dimension of the duration of a test item on the computer screen. The target pictures and the four options of pictures or distracters were counterbalanced and introduced to participants in random order. Each test item was timed for a maximum of one minute to appear on the computer screen after which the next item would appear immediately if the participant did not select an answer. The time needed to complete this test was 56 minutes (i.e., 54 minutes for the actual test and 2 minutes for the two trial exercises). Participants would get one point for each item answered correctly and a zero point for each item answered incorrectly. The maximum possible score on this instrument was 54 out of 54.

This instrument was further refined by obtaining the correlation of each item with the total score to remove from the final analysis any negative or weak test item that might negatively affect the coefficient (alpha) level. Results revealed 46 items to correlate significantly with the total score. The correlation ranged from .21 to .53. The correlation of the non-significant items ranged from .01 to .19. One item correlated negatively with the total score ($r = -.01$). This item was from the physics domain and related to gravity. This item was deleted from final analyses. The gravity or the act of falling was covered by another item in the physics domain but a different context. The significantly correlated items (i.e., $n = 46$) yielded a reliability coefficient (alpha) of .81. The 53 items, after excluding the negative item, yielded a reliability coefficient (alpha) of .79. Consequently, the 53 items were used to analyze the data since taking out the non-significant items did not improve significantly the test reliability level.

Procedures

The administration of the three tools was conducted in different locations and supervised by a data collector. Unlike the metacognitive instrument, the Mooney and the Raven Scales were administered in a group setting. Directions and instructions were verbalized orally regarding how participants should mark their responses on the answer sheets designed for the Mooney and the Raven scales.

Administering the Mooney tool in paper format took approximately one hour fifteen minutes a session without a break with a total of four sessions. Items were read aloud to all participants. Administering the Raven measure to participants was completed in four sessions each of which lasted about 50 minutes. As the case with the previous research, there was no time limit to respond to the Mooney or Raven instruments. Times stated signify the maximum time that participants took to complete the last item on the measures. Collecting the data on metacognition started by giving each participant two-trial test items. The first item presented on the computer screen was a picture of an apple and the four options of two kittens, three bananas, an open book, and a robot. Participants were requested to point to the option that was related to or matched with the target picture. The second trial was presenting a target picture of a red circle and the options of three red triangles and a red circle. Participants were asked to point to the shape that was related to or matched with the target picture. In both training exercises, the data collector used the mouse to click on the option that the participants had chosen. When the participants finished the two exercises, they began to take the actual test. Entering the participants' choices into the computer was conducted by the data collector to control for unnecessary time variations and to avoid inconsistent data entry or unintended answers that could not be reversed.

FINDINGS

A preliminary analysis of 2 (Normally and Low-achieving Participants) X 2 (Gender: Males and Females) Analysis of Variance (ANOVA) was performed to find if there were significant differences among participants on the 11 Mooney subscales (see Table 1).

Table 1. Two-way ANOVA using group membership and gender on the Mooney's 11 subscales

Study variables	Mean Square	df df error	F	Partial Eta Squared
1. HPD				
Group Membership	.306	1 84	1.028	.012
Gender	.030	1 84	.102	.001
Group Membership X Gender	1.135	1 84	3.810	.043
2. FLE				
Group Membership	.009	1 84	.033	.001
Gender	.027	1 84	.103	.001
Group Membership X Gender	.241	1 84	.907	.011
3. SRA				
Group Membership	.377	1 84	2.272	.026
Gender	2.049	1 84	12.356***	.128
Group Membership X Gender	.011	1 84	.067	.001
4. SPR				
Group Membership	.094	1 84	.466	.006
Gender	.681	1 84	3.390	.039
Group Membership X Gender	.006	1 84	.029	.001
5. PPR	.181	1 84	.835	.010
Group Membership	.091	1 84	.421	.005
Gender	4.04	1 84	1.861	.022
Group X Gender				
6. CSM				
Group Membership	3.322	1 84	13.122***	.135
Gender	1.741	1 84	6.876*	.076
Group Membership X Gender	.917	1 84	3.623	.041
7. MR				
Groups Membership	1.280	1 84	7.094**	.078
Gender	.409	1 84	2.265	.026
Groups Membership X Gender	1.636	1 84	9.065**	.097

Table 1. (Continued)

Study variables	Mean Square	df df error	F	Partial Eta Squared
8. ASW Group Membership				
Gender	.686	1 84	2.528	.029
Group Membership	.987	1 84	3.634	.041
X Gender	.781	1 84	2.877	.033
9. HF				
Group Membership	.024	1 84	.061	.001
Gender	.450	1 84	1.114	.013
Group Membership X Gender	.010	1 84	.024	.001
10. CTP				
Group Membership	8.335	1 84	25.323***	.232
Gender	1.296	1 84	3.938*	.045
Group Membership X Gender	.001	1 84	.003	.001
11. FVE				
Group Membership	.381	1 84	1.114	.013
Gender	.037	1 84	.108	.001
Group Membership X Gender	.741	1 84	2.164	.025

Note: * = $p < .05$; ** = $p < .01$; *** = $p < .001$; HPD = Health and Physical Development; FLE = Finance, Living Condition, and Employment; SRA = Social and Recreational Activities; SPR = Social-Psychological Relations; PPR = Personal-Psychological Relations; CSM = Courtship, Sex, and Marriage; MR = Morals and Religion; ASW = Adjustment to School Work; HF = Home and Family; CTP = Curriculum and Teaching Procedure; FVE = The Future: Vocational and Educational Procedure.

The analysis showed significant differences in four out of 11 areas. The first one was in the subscale of Social and Recreational Activities where male participants reported more concerns and difficulties compared to female participants regardless of a group membership. The second significant difference was in group membership and gender in the subscale of Courtship, Sex, and Marriage. The normally achieving participants reported more problems in this area than the low-achieving participants, and males reported more problems compared to females regardless of a group membership. The third significant difference was in the subscale of Morals and Religion in group membership and the interaction between group membership and gender. The normally achieving reported more problems (2.60), as a group, compared to the low-achieving participants (2.38); and the normally achieving females reported the most problems

(2.67) compared to the low-achieving females (2.16), males (2.57), or the normally achieving males (2.53); this explains the interaction found in this subscale (see Table 2). The last significant difference was in the subscale of Curriculum and Teaching Procedure in group membership and gender. The normally achieving group reported more problems in this area compared to the low-achieving group, and males in both groups reported more problems than females.

Table 2. Means comparisons (M) and standard deviations (SD) between the normally achieving and low-achieving males and females on the Mooney's 11 subscales

	Normally Achieving						**Low-Achieving**					
Mooney subscales	Total		Males		Females		Total		Males		Females	
	M	SD	M	SD	M	SD	M	SD	M	SD	M	SD
1. HPD	2.34	.504	2.24	.509	2.44	.494	2.47	.592	2.59	.515	2.33	.655
2. FLE	1.96	.496	1.92	.507	1.99	.496	1.98	.528	2.05	.619	1.91	.391
3. SRA	2.41	.396	2.55	.420	2.27	.320	2.29	.461	2.44	.377	2.11	.497
4. SPR	2.34	.415	2.42	.414	2.26	.409	2.29	.484	2.37	.404	2.18	.556
5. PPR	2.36	.465	2.26	.474	2.46	.443	2.27	.468	2.30	.375	2.23	.566
6. CSM	2.64	.389	2.67	.372	2.60	.410	2.27	.630	2.49	.516	2.00	.662
7. MR	2.60	.405	2.53	.404	2.67	.404	2.38	.484	2.57	.395	2.16	.494
8. ASW	2.84	.478	2.85	.486	2.83	.482	2.68	.583	2.86	.498	2.46	.612
9. HF	2.06	.698	2.12	.677	1.99	.729	2.03	.567	2.11	.561	1.94	.573
10. CTP	2.89	.471	3.02	.430	2.77	.487	2.29	.664	2.39	.656	2.16	.667
11. FVE	3.00	.463	2.93	.512	3.07	.408	2.87	.679	2.98	.601	2.75	.758

Note: * = $p < .05$, ** = $p < .01$. HPD = Health and Physical Development; FLE = Finance, Living Condition, and Employment; SRA = Social and Recreational Activities; SPR = Social-Psychological Relations; PPR = Personal-Psychological Relations; CSM = Courtship, Sex, and Marriage; MR = Morals and Religion; ASW = Adjustment to School Work; HF = Home and Family; CTP = Curriculum and Teaching Procedure; FVE = The Future: Vocational and Educational Procedure.

Mean responses and standard deviations for performances on the Mooney scale, the metacognitive test, reaction time, and the metacognitive performance divided by time are presented in Table 3. The table showed that both groups of participants reported low levels of issues and concerns; the mean response for the normally achieving participants was 2.50 and for the low achieving participants was 2.33 on a scale out of 4.00. The table showed differences in the variables derived from the metacognitive instrument in favor of the normally achieving participants.

Table 3. Means and standard deviations of the Mooney checklist, metacognitive test, reaction time, and metacognitive test scores divided by time

Student Groups		Mooney Checklist		Metacognitive Test Scores		Reaction Time in Seconds		Metacognitive Test Scores Divided by Time	
1. Total Normally Achieving	n	M	SD	M	SD	M	SD	M	SD
	42	2.50	.31	40.17	4.79	225.60	61.16	29.79	10.51
Males	21	2.52	.32	39.95	4.84	247.67	62.60	26.05	10.16
Females	21	2.48	.31	40.38	4.84	203.52	52.22	33.53	9.68
2. Total Low Achieving	46	2.33	.39	35.89	7.42	261.46	91.96	22.63	9.33
Males	25	2.45	.31	35.36	7.55	241.88	68.40	23.36	8.41
Females	21	2.19	.44	36.52	7.38	284.76	111.20	21.76	10.47

Four separate 2 (Normally Achieving and Low-Achieving) X 2 (Gender: Males and Females) Analysis of Variances were performed to determine if there were significant differences in performance on the four dependent variables reported in Table 3. These ANOVA analyses are reported in Table 4. The first analysis was performed to determine if there were significant differences in the total score of the Mooney scale. The result showed that the normally achieving participants, as a group, reported more problems and that males, regardless of group membership, reported more concerns and issues compared to females. The second analysis showed that the normally achieving group performed higher on the metacognitive test compared to the low-achieving group. The third analysis showed that the normally achieving participants took significantly less reaction time than the low-achieving group; and the significant interaction between the group membership and gender is determined by whether or not males and females were in low-achieving or normally achieving groups (e.g., low-achieving females taking the longest reaction time compared to normally achieving females - see Table 3). The last analysis showed the normally achieving group obtaining significantly higher metacognitive scores when divided by reaction time, and the performance of males and females is determined by their group membership (e.g., normally achieving females obtained the highest score compared to the lowest score obtained by the low-achieving females; this result, along with the performance of males in both groups, explains the interaction found in this analysis).

Table 4. Two-way ANOVA using group membership and gender on the outcome variables of Mooney checklist (MC), metacognitive test (MT), reaction time (RT), and metacognitive test scores divided by reaction time (MTRT)

Outcome variables	Mean Square	df	df error	F	Partial Eta Squared
1. MC					
Group Membership	.680	1	84	5.632*	.063
Gender	.502	1	84	4.157*	.047
Group Membership X Gender	.275	1	84	2.274	.026
2. MT					
Group Membership	390.438	1	84	9.655**	.103
Gender	13.867	1	84	.343	.004
Group Membership X Gender	2.956	1	84	.073	.001
3. RT					
Group Membership	31133.146	1	84	5.310*	.059
Gender	8.695	1	84	.001	.001
Group Membership X Gender	41416.535	1	84	7.064**	.078
4. MTRT					
Group Membership	1141.813	1	84	12.250***	.127
Gender	188.956	1	84	2.027	.024
Group Membership X Gender	450.311	1	84	4.831*	.054

Note: * = $p < .05$; ** = $p < .01$; *** = $p < .001$.

Pearson Product-Moment Correlations were conducted to find significant associations between responses to the Mooney scale, the metacognitive test, reaction time, the metacognitive test scores divided by reaction time, gender, age, IQ, language, and math (see Table 5). Results showed significant negative correlations between scores on the Mooney scale, reaction time, language, and math. It appears that a high score on the

Mooney was associated significantly with less reaction time on the metacognitive measure and lower grades in language and math; the performances on the two academic subjects were significantly correlated with each other; and language correlated significantly but negatively with the age variable, meaning that older participants got lower grades in this subject area. Table 5 showed a significant association between performances on the IQ test, the metacognitive test, and the metacognitive test scores divided by mean reaction time. Participants with high IQs obtained high scores on these two dependent variables. The table also showed that the association between responses on the Mooney scale and the metacognitive test scores divided by time almost reached the significant level (r=.20; p=.07). It revealed significant positive associations between participants' age, on the one hand, and their metacognitive test scores and metacognitive test scores divided by time, on the other hand. Older participants obtained better scores on these two variables compared to the younger ones. The table showed that females (with mean age = 16.94 years) were older than males (with mean age = 16.22) with negatively significant correlation of -.27.

Table 5. Pearson product-moment correlations of the Mooney scale, metacognitive test (MT), reaction time (RT), metacognitive test scores divided by reaction time (MTRT), gender, age, IQ, language, and math variables

Variables	1	2	3	4	5	6	7	8	9
1. Mooney (N=88)	1.00								
2. MT (N=88)	.10	1.00							
3. RT (N=88)	-.28**	-.01	1.00						
4. MTRT (N=88)	.20	.53**	-.76**	1.00					
5. Gender (N=88)	.21	-.08	.01	-.15	1.00				
6. Age (N=88)	.07	.26*	-.13	.22*	-.27*	1.00			
7. IQ (N=88)	-.04	.38**	-12	.26*	.16	-.01	1.00		
8. Language (N=88)	-.28**	-.01	-.09	.12	-.18	-.23*	-.03	1.00	
9. Math (N=88)	-.24*	.02	-.04	.08	-.17	-.15	.07	.72**	1.00

Note: * = p < .05, ** = p < .01.

Based on the results reported in the correlation table 5, Analysis of Covariance (ANCOVA) was performed to find significant differences between the two groups of participants on the Mooney scale when controlling for the effect of reaction time, language, and math. This analysis was required to show if significant differences existed between the two participating groups solely on the Mooney scale when controlling for the influencing variables. The ANCOVA analysis showed that the reaction time covariate was significant, $F(1, 81) = 5.564$, $p <.001=.02$ (partial $\eta 2 =.06$). The language, $F(1, 81) = 1.457$, $p =.23$ (partial $\eta 2 = .02$), and the math, $F(1, 81) = .211$, $p =.65$ (partial $\eta 2 = .01$), covariates were not significant. Differences between the two groups were not significant, $F(1, 81) = 1.034$, $p =.312$ (partial $\eta 2 = .01$). The gender variable was not significant, $F(1, 81) = 2.643$, $p = .108$ (partial $\eta 2 = .03$), nor was the interaction between the participants and the gender variables, $F(1, 81) = .204$, $p = .653$ (partial $\eta 2 = .01$).

Multivariate Analysis of Covariance (MANCOVA) was also performed to find significant differences between the two groups of participants on the metacognitive test, in reaction time, and on the metacognitive test scores divided by time. Participants' age, performance on the Mooney scale, and the IQ scores were all used as covariates because they correlated significantly with one or more of the three dependent variables; and the normally achieving participants were significantly older than the low achieving volunteers by 1.03 years, $F(1, 86) = 14.479$, $p <.001$.

The MANCOVA analysis revealed that the age covariate was not significant, Hotelling's $F(3, 79) = 2.232$, $p = .09$ (partial $\eta 2 = .08$); the Mooney scale covariate was significant, Hotelling's $F(3,79) = 2.885$, $p < .04$ (partial $\eta 2 = .10$); the IQ covariate was significant, Hotelling's $F(3, 79) = 4.326$, $p < .01$ (partial $\eta 2 = .14$). The results revealed that the difference in performance based on group membership was not significant, $F(3, 79) = .567$, $p = .64$ (partial $\eta 2 = .02$); the gender variable was not significant, $F(3, 79) = 2.279$, $p = .09$ (partial $\eta 2 = .08$). The interaction between participants' groups and the gender variable was not significant, $F(3, 79) = 2.346$, $p = .08$ (partial $\eta 2 = .08$).

DISCUSSION

This study explored whether QoL (as measured by the Mooney scale), metacognition, and IQ were significantly associated with each other. It was also intended to find whether or not significant differences would be found between the performances of normally and low-achieving groups on the metacognitive test, in reaction time, on the metacognitive test scores divided by time, and on the Mooney scale when controlling for the effect of all influencing variables. It was hypothesized that significant relationships would be found between the measures employed; and that no significant differences would exist between the two participating groups when controlling for the effect of contributing variables.

Analyses showed no significant differences between the normally achieving and low- achieving participants in seven out of eleven subscales, and when there were significant differences it was either the male participants reported more problems compared to females or that the normally achieving reported more problems than the low-achieving participants. This means that there are more similarities than differences between the two groups on the Mooney scale, and the few differences appeared could be attributed to the different curriculum studied and to the heterogeneity of the low-achieving group.

The results showed a significant negative correlation between the metacognitive test scores divided by time and reaction time itself, meaning that long reaction time was associated with low scores in metacognition. Results also showed a significant positive correlation between the metacognitive test scores and test scores divided by time, indicating that when test scores were high test scores divided by reaction time were also high. Furthermore, there were significant negative correlations between responses on the Mooney scale and achievements in the two subject areas of language and math. It appeared that academic achievement was a significant contributing element to the problems reported on the Mooney scale, an indication of the relationship between school achievement and life satisfaction for the participants involved in this study. While no research has been found on this topic using similar groups of participants with similar characteristics, literature pointed to the possible connection between QoL and academic achievement (1, 32).

The effect of IQ and responses on the Mooney scale appeared to be significant in the form of covariates; this was apparent when examining differences between the two groups of participants on the metacognitive test, in reaction time, and on the metacognitive test divided by time, a suggestion that they seemed to affect each other. The lack of direct significant correlation between the IQ scores and responses on the Mooney scale was contrary to the hypothesis stated in this study and to the result reported on normal hearing and D/HH individuals (1). This particular outcome warrants elaborations. Further examination of the data showed (when analyses were performed separately on each group of participants) that the IQ of normally achieving participants correlated significantly but negatively, as anticipated, with the Mooney scale ($r=-.32$; $p < .04$); this was contrary to the IQ of low-achieving participants ($r=-.08$; $p=.593$) even though both correlations were in the negative direction. Also, reaction time correlated significantly but negatively with the Mooney scale ($r=-.33$; $p < .03$) for the low-achieving group; this means that long reaction time was significantly associated with low problems on the Mooney scale, unlike the case with normally achieving participants ($r = -04$; $p =.78$), although both correlations were in the same direction. In addition, the IQ score was significantly but negatively associated with the age variable for the low-achieving group ($r= - .35$; $p < .02$) but not for the normally achieving participants ($r = -.22$; $p = .17$). This pattern of responses had been obtained probably due to the heterogeneity of the low-achieving group in terms of abilities and characteristics.

Additional and viable explanations could also be provided to shed light on the performance of the low-achieving participants. The lack of significant association between the IQ and the responses on the Mooney scale could be due to the social and financial supports that they have been receiving from the family and government alike which might have impacted their QoL. This group has been protected by the special education law titled The Right of Individuals with Disabilities - Act No. 8. (33) to guard their rights, to provide them with needed services, to guarantee equal opportunities, and to prevent discriminations based on disabilities in social, economic, health, learning, cultural, and recreational cares and welfares (34, 35). Without outside assistance, these individuals would have to rely on their mental ability as a resort to improve their QoL which, in this case, could become associated with IQ.

Another concurrent and viable explanation could be the inconsistency of responses of the low-achieving group due to the lack of accurately estimated answers to the orally presented problems. As stated earlier, it could be that the diversity of the low-achieving group contributed to this result. This group might have failed to balance its responses to the presented items on the Mooney scale to reflect its situations, actual abilities, and available opportunities to a degree that its performance did not correlate significantly with the IQ scores like the case with the normally achieving individuals. This might be a plausible explanation when considering that the low-achievement group was formed of individuals with various characteristics and traits; that is, it was not uniquely defined or being considered a proper group in special education based on multiple diagnostic criteria; it actually consisted of participants with low-achievement irrespective of the exact factors, causes, or hidden disabilities compounded with inadequate assessment and diagnosis, unlike the normally achieving or D/HH individuals (1, 16). Overall, future research may explore this matter in-depth to determine if the lack of significant association is a unique characteristic of this group or that the group should be more accurately defined based on the causes of their low-achievement.

It is to note in the case of the low-achievement group that no significant relationship between IQ and QoL (as reflected in responses on the Mooney scale) was contrary to their performance in metacognition. The metacognitive test scores were significantly correlated with IQ, meaning that high metacognitive scores were associated with high IQs; and the metacognitive test scores divided by time were significantly associated with the metacognitive test scores by which showing that high performance in one was accompanied with enhanced performance in the other; this result was contrary to the one obtained regarding reaction time where longer reaction time was negatively associated with low performance on the metacognitive test score divided by time. This outcome was expected and showed the negative impact of time on performance (27).

The results also showed that the performance on the metacognitive test was significantly influenced by the age and IQ variables; high IQ scores were accompanied by high performance on the metacognitive test and older participants performed better than younger ones. Previous research conducted on normally hearing and on D/HH participants supported this result (1, 27).

Considering QoL is a fluid concept, this present research suggests that the individual's metacognitive ability, as conceptualized in this current study and others (36), should not be overlooked when approaching QoL. Also, while the result of this study did not show that IQ correlated significantly with QoL for the low-achieving participants, the author still considers IQ to play a role in skill acquisitions and skill deficits of all individuals, with and without disabilities. The level of IQ determines the type and/or the nature of tasks to be accomplished and the environment where it is deemed crucial to do so. This point has been tacitly recognized by Brown and Brown (13) when stating that choices, as a fundamental principle in the QoL of individuals with intellectual disabilities, may not be adopted but adapted based on the developmental stage of the individuals and drawn from the assessment data.

It is to emphasize that the QoL index could change over time from low to high and vice versa because it deals with self-evaluation within one's culture in which opportunities are provided, offered, stumbled with, or even missed. These opportunities form and shape the QoL of any individual. Although raw responses on the Mooney scale appeared not that high, negative issues should be dealt with efficiently and professionally for both groups by eliminating social and environmental barriers including discriminations, symptoms of stress and other risk factors, and performing effective teaching practices to enhance achievement and improve QoL.

Whether the problems are actual or perceived, they could not be addressed in isolation from significantly contributing factors such as IQ (as the case with the normally achieving participants) and school achievement. These factors should be examined in depth in future studies since they have a moderating effect on behaviors and social adjustment and on the reported problems as seen in this study and others (1).

Also, many of the issues reported are not uncommon and could be found everywhere. The necessity is to identify them to provide needed interventions by collecting data through rating scales, clinical interviews, observations, and standardized tests.

CONCLUSION

This study is exploratory in nature. It showed that school achievement in math and language was significantly but negatively associated with performance on the Mooney scale. What needs to be examined further is the result concerning the IQ and performance on the Mooney scale. Current results showed that both measures were significant covariates when examining differences between participants on the metacognitive instrument but the IQ failed to correlate significantly with performance on the Mooney scale. Did the problem rest on overestimating and exaggerating responses to the issues addressed by the Mooney scale on the part of the low-achieving participants or did the social support have made that much of a difference in their lives? Or did the issue rest on group heterogeneity? Only future research could answer these questions by conducting similar work on QoL using participants who are low-achieving and who have similar traits like the ones reported in this study.

Future research may address the issues raised in this study and recruit a larger sample of participants with full data related to IQ and school achievement. It is believed that a clearer picture would also be obtained when collecting the aforementioned data and including in the research participants with a designated special needs like deafness in addition to normally achieving and high achieving participants. This research might show conformity, dichotomy, or spectrum of QoL levels among groups of individuals living in the same community where QoL is easily influenced by social and environmental variables. This suggested research may also explore differences among various instruments that measure QoL through self-reporting and self-perceptions, on the one hand, and the relationship with IQ and with metacognition, on the other hand.

Acknowledgments

Data collected for this study during working as an Associate Professor of Special Education in the Department of Educational Psychology, College of Education, Kuwait University, State of Kuwait.

References

[1] Al-Hilawani Y. Hearing and deaf and hard-of-hearing: A comparison on metacognition, the Mooney problem checklist, IQ, and gender. Volta Rev 2016;16(1):5-28.

[2] Shelp EE. Born to die? Deciding the fate of critically ill newborns. New York: Free Press, 1986.

[3] Sparks RC. To treat or not to treat: Bioethics and the handicapped newborn. New York: Paulist Press, 1988.

[4] Wolfensberger W. The extermination of handicapped people in World War II Germany. Ment Retard 1981;19:1-7.

[5] Hollander R. Euthanasia and mental retardation: Suggesting the unthinkable. Ment Retard 1989;27(2):53-61.

[6] Coulter DL. Beyond Baby Doe: Does infant transplantation justify euthanasia? J Assoc Persons Severe Handicaps 1988;13(2):71-5.

[7] Lusthaus, E. Involuntary euthanasia and current attempts to define persons with mental retardation as less than human. Ment Retard 1985;23(3):148-15.

[8] Individuals with Disabilities Education Improvement Act-IDEA. Public Law 108-446- 108th Congress, 2004.

[9] Kuhse H, Singer P. Should the baby live? The problem of handicapped infants. Oxford: Oxford University Press, 1985.

[10] World Health Organization. WHOQOL measuring quality of life. The World Health Organization Quality of Life Instruments (WHOQOL-100 and WHOQOL-BREF). WHOQOL Group. Programme on Mental Health Division of Mental Health and Prevention of Substance Abuse. Geneva: WHO, 1997. URL: http://www.who.int/mental_health/media/68.pdf.

[11] The WHOQOL group. The World Health Organization Quality of Life Assessment (WHOQOL): Position paper from the World Health Organization. Soc Sci Med 1995;41: 1403-09.

[12] Cummins RA. Moving from the quality of life concept to a theory. J Intellect Disabil Res 2005;49 699-706.

[13] Brown RI, Brown I. The application of quality of life. J Intellect Disabil Res 2005;49: 718-27.

[14] Verdugo MA, Schalock RL, Keith KD, Stancliffe RJ. Quality of life and its measurement: Important principles and guidelines. J Intellect Disabil Res 2005;49:707–17.

[15] Lusthaus, E. Euthanasia of persons with severe handicaps: Refuting the rationalizations. J Assoc Persons Severe Handicaps 1985;10(2) 87-94.

[16] Al-Hilawani, Y. Educational practices and services for students with learning disabilities in Oman: Proposed guidelines. J Int Assoc Specl Educ, in press.

[17] Sternberg RJ, Grigorenko E, Bundy DA. The predictive value of IQ. Merrill-Palmer Quart 2001;47:1-41.

[18] Nota L, Ferrari L, Soresi S, Wehmeyer M. Self-determination, social abilities and the quality of life of people with intellectual disability. J Intellect Disabil Res 2007;51:850-65.

[19] Brown AL. Knowing when, where, and how to remember: A problem of metacognition. In: Glaser R, ed. Advances in instructional psychology, vol. 1. Hillsdale NJ: Erlbaum, 1978:77-165.

[20] Flavell JH. Metacognitive aspects of problem-solving. In: Resnick LB, ed. The nature of intelligence. Hillsdale NJ: Lawrence Erlbaum, 1976:231-5.

[21] Al-Hilawani Y. Measuring students' metacognition in real-Life situations. Am Ann Deaf 2003;148:233-42.

[22] Al-Hilawani Y, Easterbrooks SR, Marchant GJ. Metacognitive ability from a theory-of-mind perspective: A cross-cultural study of students with and without hearing loss. Am Ann Deaf 2002;147:38–47.

[23] Al-Hilawani Y, Abdullah AA. Measuring metacognition and reaction time: Further findings on the performances of general education, low-achieving, and institutionally raised students. J Int Spec Needs Educ 2010;13:1-13.

[24] Meichenbaum DA. Cognitive-behavioral perspective on intelligence. Intelligence 1980; 4:271-83.

[25] Veenman M, Wilhelm P, Beishuizen JJ. The relation between intellectual and metacognitive skills from a developmental perspective. Learn Instruction 2004;14:89-109.

[26] Al-Hilawani Y, Dashti F, Abdullah A. Measuring metacognition: A prospect for objective assessment. Volta Rev 2008;108:139-54.

[27] Al-Hilawani Y. Metacognition and group differences: A comparative study. Exceptionality Spec Educ J 2014;22: 73-89.

[28] Raven JC, Court J H, Raven J. Manual for Raven's standard progressive matrices. Oxford: Oxford Psychologists Press, 1996.

[29] Mooney RL, Gordon LV. The Mooney Problem Checklists. New York: Psychological Corporation, 1950.

[30] The WHOQOL GROUP. The World Health Organization Quality of Life Assessment (WHOQOL): Development and general psychometric properties. Soc Sci Med 1998;46: 1569-85.

[31] Wellman HM., Gelman SA. Cognitive development: Foundational theories of core domains. Annu Rev Psychol 1992;43:337-75.

[32] Dilley J. Research Review: School-based health interventions and academic achievement 2009. URL: http://here.doh.wa.gov/materials/research-review-school-based-health-interventions-and-academic-achievement/12_HealthAcademic_E09L.pdf.

[33] The right of individuals with disabilities – Act No. 8. State of Kuwait, 2010.

[34] Al-Hilawani Y. The lost Kuwait initiative: The failure has come from within. J Int Spec Needs Educ 2011;14(1):42-8.

[35] Al-Hilawani Y. Perspectives and reviews on deafness in the State of Kuwait and the United Arab Emirates. In: Moores DF, Miller MS, eds. Deaf people around the world: Educational and social perspectives. Washington DC: Gallaudet University Press, 2009: 119-32.

[36] Al-Hilawani Y. Visual analyses and discriminations: One approach to measuring students' metacognition. Am Ann Deaf 2006;151:16-24.

In: Intellectual Disability
Editors: Ariel Tenenbaum et al.
ISBN: 978-1-53617-866-1

Chapter 6

HOW FAMILY CARERS SUPPORT PROFOUNDLY INTELLECTUALLY DISABLED PERSONS IN DECISION MAKING: A LITERATURE REVIEW

Ruth Ryan**, PhD
Department of Nursing and Midwifery, Faculty of Education and Health Sciences, University of Limerick, Ireland

ABSTRACT

This chapter presents a literature review, an element of a larger study, exploring Irish family carers' experiences of supporting person, living with profound intellectual and multiple disabilities, in decision making. An eclectic approach to the review was warranted as little empirical evidence was found. In all 23 policies/reports are reviewed in addition to 25 theoretical and research papers. Review findings are presented in three sections; 1) General information and background to supporting decision

* Corresponding Author: Ruth Ryan, RNID, RNT, PhD, Lecturer, Address: Department of Nursing and Midwifery, Faculty of Education and Health Sciences, University of Limerick, Ireland. E-mail: Ruth.Ryan@ul.ie.

making 2) Models of 'supporting decision making' and 3) Challenges within a "Principle Based Concept." The main contribution of this literature review is the provision of a baseline to support forthcoming research in the area of SDM and secondly to highlight tensions within implementing what appears initially as a normative and simplistic concept.

INTRODUCTION

A commitment to incorporate rights based approaches to support disabled persons to live a full and ordinary life exists (1-4) with families in Ireland, similar to other countries, remaining the main providers of support for people with intellectual disabilities (ID) (5). This paper presents one element, the literature review, of a research project which is 'exploring Irish family carers experiences of supporting person, living with profound intellectual and multiple disabilities (PIMD), in decision making'. It is well acknowledged that family carers in general and specifically family carers caring and supporting persons, living with PIMD, are recognised as the main source of support for people who require help to live in their own homes with research in this area blooming in the past three decades (6-10). A wave of change has bestowed these families in terms of normalisation and personalising supports, social structures ensuring accessibility and provision of public services for all, and now moving into the 21st Century the concept of "supporting decision making" purporting to facilitate disabled persons in the process of individual empowered choice making. Reflecting international views this paper aims to explore these changes from an Irish context.

BACKGROUND

In general, family caring literature focuses primarily on carers of older persons, family carers and persons, living with dementia, and newer insights are addressing "young carers" (6, 11, 12) with few studies addressing this specific needs of family carers supporting the intellectually disabled (ID) population (13). It is acknowledged that family caregivers play a vital key role in supporting disabled people in their health, wellbeing and participation (14) yet challenges in this role have arisen and more so in current discussions in relation to the United Nations (UN) Conventions on the Rights of Persons with Disabilities (CRPD) understanding of supporting decision making (SDM).

'Support' is a normative and common word that encompasses many meanings. The American Association of Intellectual and Developmental Disabilities (AAIDD) define support as a psychological construct referring to the pattern and intensity of resources and strategies that promote personal development and enhance functioning that a person requires participating in activities associated with normative human functioning (17) and the personalisation agenda becomes interwoven with decision making (18). Family carers engage, intensely, in promoting personal development, thereby enhancing their sons and daughters engagement in human functioning and therefore have a major role to play in supporting persons, living with PIMD, in decision-making.

As an emerging legal concept, SDM is a term advocated by the UN CRPD and represents an emergent legal status that will be of benefit, in particular, to people with significant or 'profound' intellectual, psychosocial, and communication disabilities (15, 16). The essence of SDM is to enable people to maintain full legal capacity (both recognition of rights and capacity to exercise those rights) while availing themselves of legally recognised access to supports (19, 20). In this manner, persons, living with profound intellectual and multiple disabilities (PIMD), therefore would be regarded as independent persons rejecting historical notions of disability and their assumptions of 'lacking capacity' to make decisions. Supported decision-making is thus presented here, with the assumptions and understandings of the UN CRPD Handbook for Parliamentarians on the Convention, as:

> 'Those assisting a person may communicate the individual's intentions to others or help him/her understand the choices at hand. They

may help others to realise that a person with significant disabilities is also a person with a history, interest and aims in life, and is someone capable of exercising his/her legal capacity' pp.X.

Family carers report that the time, effort, resources and strategies in supporting persons, living with PIMD, to promote personal development and function, is considerable (21). Balancing legislation and policy to complement and enhance family carers' roles to maximise their ability to care for their family member/relative is important yet challenging. Some disability theorist suggest the word 'carer' 'care' and 'caring for' in the context of supporting persons with disabilities is haunted by the spectres of institutionalisation, medicalisation and paternalistic charities which characterises 'caring for' as a complex form of oppression systematically marginalising people with disabilities and therefore terms such as support, personal assistance are preferable (22). Article 12(3) of the CRPD specifically references State parties role in providing support as follows:

States parties shall take appropriate measures to provide access by persons with disabilities to the support they may require in exercising their legal capacity.

It has been argued however, that policies that support carers could be interpreted as reinforcing or perpetuating the oppression and dependency of person with disabilities as tensions arise between policies to support carers and policies aimed at promoting choice and control for persons with disabilities (23). This can be due in part by the disjointed approach of government departments in addressing health and social policies, and disconnect between policy makers and different government departments. From an Irish perspective, the first Irish Carers Strategy was produced in 2012 'The National Carers' Strategy Recognised, Supported, Empowered' (10) recognises that carers are the 'backbone of care provision' in Ireland.

IRISH CARERS STRATEGY RECOGNISED, SUPPORTED EMPOWERED

Like most countries the Irish government recognises how our ageing population and medical advances in relation to disability and chronic illness will result in more people, of all ages, with longer term and complex care needs requiring care and being cared for in the community in the future (10). Therefore recognition of general and specific needs of carers requires a strategic and co-ordinated approach. The strategy recognised "Supported empowered" has four national goals which are to:

- Recognise the value and contribution of carers and promote their inclusion in decisions relating to the person they are caring for
- Support carers to manage their physical, mental and emotional health and well-being
- Support carers to care with confidence through the provision of adequate information, training, services and supports
- Empower carers to participate as fully as possible in economic and social life

The national carers' strategy espouses to be interconnected and not exist in isolation but an integral part of the government's broader social inclusion including the National disability strategy (1) and the National housing strategy for people with a disability (24).

Combined with this strategic governmental support many essential supports available for Irish carers and care recipients are provided by non-governmental 'voluntary' organisations which represent the interests of carers and care recipients at a local and national level, such as Carers Association, Parents and Friends Associations, National Parents and Siblings Alliance, Inclusion Ireland and Care Alliance Ireland. In addition to providing services (social services, training, information etc.), they advocate on behalf of carers and play a central role in ensuring that their needs are articulated to those with responsibility for the development of policies that directly or indirectly impact on carers; structures similar to other countries. The integrated approach to supporting carers and care recipient has benefits, and evidence suggests that this integrated approach in partnership with families identifies their specific needs so that they are able to access and be provided with support they need (25), however the print version of 'what is there' is often different to the reality of experience of recipients (26).

Aim and objective of review

The literature review aims to identify the evidence base related to how family carers support persons, living with PIMD, in decision making. The purpose of the review is to ascertain existing empirical data that may contribute to further understanding the concept, processes and structures of supporting decision making. Specific questions answered were as follows:

- What is known about how family carers' support persons, living with a PIMD, in decision making?
- Considerations when involving people, living with a profound intellectual and multiple disability, in decision-making

OUR SEARCH

A multi-method search strategy was used, including an electronic database search and manual search. The review process involved problem identification, search of current literature, evaluation of recovered data and analysis informed by Moher et al, PRISMA standards for reporting systematic reviews (27).

Search terms

In order to find appropriate literature an important feature of the literature review relates to that of problem identification. The PICO process is a technique used in evidence based practice to frame and answer a clinical or health care related question. The PICO acronym stands for. P – patient, problem or population. I – intervention.

Table 1. Pico table

Population:	**'Family Carers' OR 'Family Caregivers' OR 'Family Caregiver'**
Intervention:	'Support' OR' involve' OR 'provision of choice' OR SDM OR Supporting decision making OR decision making AND 'PIMD' OR 'person with PIMD' OR 'profound intellectual disability' OR 'profound intellectual and multiple disability'
Comparison:	N/A
Outcomes:	Decision making

Table 1 Pico Table for this stage appropriate search terms are required therefore the following descriptions demonstrate meaning of such concepts.

Family carer

A carer is someone who is providing an ongoing significant level of care to a person who is in need of that care in the home due to illness or disability or frailty as described in the Irish Carers Strategy (Irish Carers Strategy pg. 8)

Supports

Resources and strategies that promote personal development and enhance functioning' (17) in addition to the UN CRPD (2006) the Handbook for

Parliamentarians on the Convention describes supported decision making as:

> Those assisting a person may communicate the individual's intentions to others or help him/her understand the choices at hand. They may help others to realize that a person with significant disabilities is also a person with a history, interest and aims in life, and is someone capable of exercising his/her legal capacity.

Decision making

A capacity to understand and balance the necessary information and to communicate a choice (28).

Person with a PIMD

A person with profound intellectual and multiple disability have extremely delayed intellectual and social functioning, may have limited ability to engage verbally, but respond to cues within their environment (e.g., familiar voice, touch, gestures), often require those who are familiar with them to interpret their communication intent, frequently have an associated medical condition which may include neurological problems, and physical or sensory impairments. They have the chance to engage and to achieve their optimum potential in a highly structured environment with constant support with an individualized relationship with a carer (29).

Including 'Family carers' OR 'Family caregivers' OR 'Family caregiver' relates to MeSh terms. MeSh is as the National Library of Medicine's (NLM) controlled vocabulary thesaurus. It consists of sets of terms naming descriptors in a hierarchical structure that permits searching at various levels of specificity. The MeSH thesaurus is used by NLM for indexing articles from 5,400 of the world's leading biomedical journals for the MEDLINE/PubMED database. Therefore utilising MeSh terms has the ability to include a wider range of hits. The following terms were identified as shown in Table 2.

Table 2. Search terms MeSh browser

MeSH Heading	Concept View	Entry Term
Caregivers	'Persons who provide care to those who need supervision or assistance in illness or disability. They may provide the care in the home, in a hospital, or in an institution. Although caregivers include trained medical, nursing, and other health personnel, the concept also refers to parents, spouses, or other family members, friends, members of the clergy, teachers, social workers, fellow patients' This review refers to family carers only	Care Givers Carers Family Caregivers
PIMD		No term found
Support		No term found
Decision making	'The process of making a selective intellectual judgment when presented with several complex alternatives consisting of several variables, and usually defining a course of action or an idea'	Decision making

Keywords were inputted into the databases PubMed, Medline, Cumulative Index to Nursing and Allied Health Literature, PsycInfo, AMED and limited to peer reviewed journals from January 2000–November 2014. Electronic searches of Web of Science and Cochrane Library were also conducted for articles published from January 1990-November 2014. Boolean phrases 'OR' 'AND' allowed a clear focused search strategy comprising of; 'Family Carers' OR 'Family Caregivers' OR 'Family Caregiver' AND 'Support' OR 'involve' OR 'provision of choice' AND 'PIMD' OR 'person with PIMD' OR 'profound intellectual disability' OR 'profound intellectual and multiple disability' AND 'decision mak*'.

Identification of Eligible Studies

Inclusion criteria were eligible articles were studies with original data that evaluated family carers of persons with PIMD in any aspect of decision making published in English inclusive of case series and case reports (key question 1 & 2). Time limiters applied from 1990-2014.

Exclusion criteria: Commentary, abstracts, letters and editorials were excluded at this point. To summaries this approach Table 3 below outlines the stage and rationale of the systematic review approach; the results of the search;

Table 3. Systematic approach to searching literature

Stage of Systematic literature review	Decisions and rationale
Question/Problem Identification	Aim for the review; To identify the evidence base related to how family carers support persons with PIMD in decision making. *PICO application* **Population**: 'Family Carers' OR 'Family Caregivers' OR 'Family Caregiver' **Intervention**: 'Support' OR' involve' OR 'provision of choice' AND 'PIMD' OR 'person with PIMD' OR 'profound intellectual disability' OR 'profound intellectual and multiple disability' **Comparison**: N/A **Outcomes**: decision making
Search of Literature Databases used	1) PubMed (Retrieved 0) 2) CINAHL Plus with Full Text (Retrieved 0) 3) PsycARTICLES (Retrieved 0) 4) PsycINFO (Retrieved 0) 5) Web of Science (Retrieved 0) 6) Cochrane Library (Retrieved 0)

This finding while disappointing was a finding in itself. One could say this highlights 'a gap in the literature' with regard to the evidence base of family carers supporting persons with PIMD in decision making. I pondered, and guided by principles of reflection I gave this matter further consideration noted in the following reflection;

Journal reflections 1: Questioning literature review approach

> *Reflection*
>
> *While this review demonstrates sound evidence for future research in this area, I am at odds with the results. Highly regarded and extremely relevant I am not convinced of the systematic 'one approach'/'all or nothing approach' to the systematic review.*
>
> *Conscious of Gooding (2013) writings and reflect on his comments 'since the coming into force of the CRPD, activity around supported decision-making has gained a small but visible momentum in academic monographs, academic journal articles, case law, regional courts and bodies, legislative reform activity in the formation of centres and institutes, in a growing body of 'grey literature' the operation of conferences and symposia and in UN activity' Having reviewed some of the grey literature, attended the conferences and engaged in and with the UN website frequently through curiosity and knowledge development, inclusion of other sources appears just.*

Consideration of other approaches to reviewing the literature was sought noting the importance of 'grey literature'. The inclusion of a range of evidence from other sources for example professional, theoretical and practice offers potential insight into a subject matter and concurs with the move beyond the reductionist approach to research, towards a deer understanding of historical, cultural and political contexts. Wallace and Wray (30) described such a framework which they classified literature in four categories namely; Theoretical literature; Research literature; Practice literature and Policy literature (30). Such an approach complements practice and policy contributions to knowledge and was thus adopted as legitimate in the context of understanding of the families' carers' experiences supporting persons, living with PIMD, in decision making.

In gathering literature in this eclectic approach, a policy or paper had to: address family carers and person, living with PIMD, and an aspect of SDM, be publicly available or archived and be published between 1990 and 2014. Irish and English policies and legislation impacting on health and social care departments were reviewed, in addition to the UN CRPD. Google Scholar, a freely available search tool was utilised. Terms "'decision making' AND 'family carers' AND 'profound disability' were utilised. To narrow the search, articles were reviewed by title and abstract and accepted if they addressed family carers and person, living with PIMD, and an aspect of SDM. Reference list of included papers were reviewed with the research questions in mind. This elicited a number of academic papers, governmental policies and legislation (focused on UK and Ireland). The following tables identify and summarise the main contributions of the reviewed documents. Table 4 presents a chronological synopsis of key Irish and UK Practice and Policy Reports related to 'family carers' 'PIMD' and some aspect of 'supporting decision making' from the year 2000 onwards. Inclusion of the UK policy was based upon our close alignment to the UK, and lessons learned from our nearest neighbour. In all, 23 policies/reports are described.

Table 5 presents a summary of the aim, methodologies and main findings of theoretical and research literature pertaining to supporting persons with PIMD in decision making albeit form healthcare professional, paid carers or teachers perspectives in all 25 articles reviewed.

Table 4. Practice and policy literature reviewed

	Year	Policy/Report	Country	Focus of Policy
1	2001	Valuing People A New Strategy for Learning Disability for the 21st Century,	United Kingdom	Introduction of four key principles of Rights, Independence, Choice, Inclusion to health and social care services and introduction of funding (50 million) on an annual basis. Aim to Shift culture of dependency and charity status of persons with ID.
2	2004	National Disability Strategy	Ireland	The Strategy, first of its kind in Ireland, aims to underpin the participation of people with disabilities (physical, intellectual and sensory) in society. Two page publication. The objective of the National Disability Strategy is to put in place legislation, policies, institutional arrangements and services to support and reinforce equal participation for people with disabilities.
3	2005	Mental Capacity Act 2005 (UK)	England and Wales	Legislation came into force in October 2007 in which a person is presumed to make their own decisions "unless all practical steps to help him (or her) to make a decision have been taken without success." A Code of Practice provides guidance and information about how the Act works in practice it should be viewed as guidance rather than instruction-. Implications for families, healthcare, legal and research practitioners.

	Year	Policy/Report	Country	Focus of Policy
4	2006	United Convention on the Rights of Persons with Disabilities (UN CRPD)	United States of America	'To promote, protect and ensure the full and equal enjoyment of all human rights and fundamental freedoms by all persons with disabilities'
5	2007	Aiming high for disabled children; better support for families	United Kingdom	Promoting the life chances of disabled children and their families though equality of opportunity, increasing involvement and inclusion in society. Three priority areas to improve outcomes for disabled children: access and empowerment, responsive services and timely support and improving quality and capacity.
6	2007	Death by Indifference	United Kingdom	Reports circumstances surrounding the death of six people with learning disabilities who died in the care of the NHS, exposing 'institutional discrimination'. Described prolonged suffering highlighting neglect and inappropriate care of these individuals. Sparked national review of standards of care.
7	2008	'Carers at the heart of 21st-century families and communities, A caring system on your side. A life of your own.'	United Kingdom	Building on from previous 'Carers A Strategy Caring for Carers' (1999) recognises the need for integrated approaches to supporting carers in their role outlining a vision that by 2018; carers will be universally recognised and valued as being fundamental to strong families and stable communities. Support will be tailored to meet individuals' needs, enabling carers to maintain a balance between their caring responsibilities and a life outside caring, whilst enabling the person they support to be a full and equal citizen.
8	2008	Healthcare for All; Report of the Independent Inquiry into access to healthcare for people with learning disabilities	United Kingdom	This inquiry found that the experiences of the families described in Mencap report 'Death by Indifference' are by no means isolated, despite a clear framework of legislation against discrimination. The Inquiry found evidence that people with learning disabilities have higher levels of unmet need and receive less effective treatment.
9	2009	Supporting Learning Disability Partnership Boards to implement the National Carers Strategy	United Kingdom	Aims to connect Learning Disability Partnership Boards and National Carers Strategy ensuring joined up approaches with any work to support carers in their local area.

Table 4. (Continued)

	Year	Policy/Report	Country	Focus of Policy
				An important document as underlying tensions between policies to support carers and policies aimed at promoting choice and control by people with ID emerge.
10	2009	Valuing People Now	United Kingdom	To 're-charge' the momentum and commitment in recognising governments support to persons with learning disabilities. Committed to undertake a three year confidential inquiry (CI) into premature deaths among the population of people with learning disabilities. A commitment to work with all families as valued partners is clearly evident in this strategy more so than the previous strategy.
11	2009	Report of the Reference Group on Multidisciplinary Services for Children aged 5 to 18 Years (completed in 2009 and approved by the HSE in 2010) (Roche et al. 2009)	Ireland	Highlighted the diversity of service provision and calls for interdisciplinary team model and 'Effective Team Working' in assessing, planning, implementing and evaluating service plan for each child.
12	2010	The National Progressing Disability Services for Children and Young People Programme (led by the HSE in partnership with the non-statutory disability organisations, Dept. of Health, Dept. of Education and Skills and associated agencies	Ireland	The vision of the programme is that each and every child or young person (5-18) with a disability will be supported to achieve their full potential through the implementation of an integrated service model that will allow children, whatever the nature of their disability, to be seen and supported as locally to their home and school as possible based on their needs. Implementation is though consultation, and reports such as the following enabling inclusive approaches to service design and delivery; Outcomes for Children and their Families (2013), Framework for Collaborative Working between Education and Health Professionals and Report on the Findings of Consultation on Outcomes Statements 2013

	Year	Policy/Report	Country	Focus of Policy
13	2010	Dignam, C. (2010) 'Second Revised Report of the Non Statutory Inquiry into the Transfer of Mr Peter McKenna to Leas Cross Nursing Home' (Dignam 2010)	Ireland	Comprehensive inquiry (at the request of the family) which focused on the decision to transfer Mr McKenna (a ward of court) from St. Michaels House to Leas cross nursing home. Mr McKenna, a client of St. Michael's House since the mid 1970's, was transferred from St. Michael's House to Leas Cross Nursing Home on the 10th October 2000. Mr McKenna died on the 22nd October 2000.
14	2010	'Raising our sights: services for adults with PIMD', A report by Jim Mansell. Tizard Learning Disability Review, 15(3), 5-12. (Mansell 2010)	England	Emphsisises the focus on ensuring meaningfully representation for people living with PIMD. To illustrate this and other prominent issues addressed in the report, accompanying you tube film were produced to disseminate and inform others, professional and public alike
15	2011	Time to Move on from Congregated Settings: A Strategy for Community Inclusion (HSE 2011)	Ireland	Identifies the mechanism of supporting the transition of each individual with disabilities identified as currently living in a congregated type setting to a more socially inclusive community integrated service over the next number of years-'nonspecific year span'
16	2011	National Housing Strategy for people with disabilities (Department of the Environment Community and Local Government 2011)	Ireland	Facilitate access, for people with disabilities, to the appropriate range of housing and related support services, delivered in an integrated and sustainable manner, which promotes equality of opportunity, individual choice and independent living, with a view to Implementation by 2016. Ambitious
17	2012	New Directions Personal Support Services for Adults with Disabilities (HSE 2012)	Ireland	This report sets out a new approach to the provision of day services for people with disabilities. Supports will be made available in natural communities offering choice and options about how to live a life of ones' choosing and how to spend ones' time. Flexible and individualised set of supports to enable each person to live a life of their choosing in accordance with their own wishes and needs is to be a minimum standard of such services.
18	2012	The National Carers Strategy: Recognised, Supported, Empowered (Department of Health 2012a)	Ireland	The first Carer's Strategy in Irish history. This Cross-Departmental Strategy acknowledges the numbers and level of commitment demonstrated by carers in the ROI.

Table 4. (Continued)

	Year	Policy/Report	Country	Focus of Policy
		Implementation of this strategy is however described on the 'cold front' as lacking (Memo 30th October 2014)		The strategy envisages family carers in care planning and decision making for those that they care for, and the promotion of supports and services to protect the physical, mental and emotional health and wellbeing of carers. Annual implementation reports concentrates on actions for the short to medium term, to be achieved on a cost neutral basis.
19	2012	The Value for Money and Policy Review of Disability Services in Ireland (Department of Health 2012b)	Ireland	Fundamental change in approach to the governance, funding and focus of the Disability Services Programme, with migration from an approach predominantly centred on group-based service delivery towards a model of person-centred and individually chosen supports. Supports to be underpinned by more effective assessing of need, allocating resources and monitoring resource use.
20	2012	Transforming Care: A National Response to Winterbourne View Hospital (UK Department of Health 2012)	United Kingdom	Reviews the scandal that unfolded at Winterbourne View exposing a culture of cruelty and crimes towards people with learning disabilities. Calls for as a matter of urgency open and positive culture in care systems. A call for leadership and cultural challenge that this scandal has exposed underpinned by listening and involving people with learning disabilities and their families
21	2013	The Confidential Inquiry into premature deaths of people with a learning disability (CIPOLD) Author; (Heslop et al. 2013)	United Kingdom	'CIPOLD investigated the sequence of events leading to all known deaths of people with disabilities (aged 4 years and older) over a 2-year period in 5 Primary Care Trust (PCT) areas of South West England; the area had a mixture of urban and rural communities and a population of 1.7m. In order to identify whether findings were specific to people with learning disabilities, the study included 58 comparator cases of adults without learning disabilities who died in the study area.
22	2013	Value for Money Implementation Framework (Department of Health 2013)	Ireland	Reflective of a change of governance structures, attitude and culture Goal 1 Full inclusion and self-determination for people with disabilities through access to the

	Year	Policy/Report	Country	Focus of Policy
				individualised personal social supports and services needed to live a fully included life in the community. Goal 2 The creation of a cost-effective, responsive and accountable system which will support the full inclusion and self-determination of people with disabilities.
23	2013	Assisted Decision Making (Capacity) Bill (2013) ...(*Assisted Decision Making (Capacity) Act* 2015)	Ireland	Long awaited Act to replace the Lunacy Act 1871 and repeals Marriage of Lunatics Act 1811. This act updates and reforms the law governing decision-making by people whose capacity may be impaired. The aim is to enable individuals to have greater autonomy in decision-making provideing a range of options for people who need support on decision-making. Reform of the law was required to enable the Irish State to ratify the UN CRPD. Also gives effect in the State to the Hague Convention on the International Protection of Adults.

Table 5. Theoretical literature reviewed

	Author(s) & Year & Journal	Country	Aim	Methodology and Design	Main Findings
1)	Browning M, Bigby C, Douglas J. Supported decision making: Understanding how its conceptual link to legal capacity is influencing the development of practice. *Research and Practice in Intellectual and Developmental Disabilities.* 2014 Jan 2;1(1):34-45.	Australia	'To help readers to understand the conceptual link between supported decision making and legal capacity and how this is influencing the development of practice'	Discursive paper	SDM is an enigmatic and ill-defined concept If developed SDM may empower and enrich the lives of people with cognitive disabilities. SDM is referred to as a process, a mechanism, a system, a framework and an end that legally recognises the process of supporting a person with their decision making. Intended to replace guardianship, an alternative legal regime to substituted

Table 5. (Continued)

	Author(s) & Year & Journal	Country	Aim	Methodology and Design	Main Findings
					decision making, complaint Article 12 UN CRPD is a philosophically driven position, embedded in human rights principles requiring a socio-contextual change.
2)	Carney T. Clarifying, operationalising, and evaluating supported decision making models. *Research and Practice in Intellectual and Developmental Disabilities*. 2014 Jan 2;1(1):46-50.	Australia	'To move from rhetoric and move to developing the research base that is so necessary to sound policymaking or law reform in the area of SDM'	Commentary/ Reports on	SDM is challenging on many fronts. Comments on 3 small scale pilot studies described (n=6 to 26) SDM with persons with ID. Meaning of SDM is uncertain and wide spectrum of models including the distinctions between "support with" decision making and "supported decision making and the relationship with legal capacity.
3)	Dept Justice and Attorney General Queensland Government, A journey towards autonomy? Supported decision making in theory and practice. A review of the literature, URL http://www.justice.qld.gov.au/__data/assets/pdf_file/0005/249404/Decision-making-support-	Australia (The Office of the Public Advocate)	As part of a research project this literature review examines the provision of decision-making support to adults with impaired decision-making capacity that interacts with the Queensland guardianship system	Literature Review (Non-Systematic)	Concept SDM poorly defined, implemented and a lack of empirical evidence. Models of SDM such as circles of support or stepped approach are elaborated upon. Concerns highlighted

	Author(s) & Year & Journal	Country	Aim	Methodology and Design	Main Findings
	for-Queenslanders-with-impaired-capacity-A-review-of-literature-March-2014.pdf last accessed November 2014				
4)	Flynn E, Arstein-Kerslake A. Legislating personhood: Realising the right to support in exercising legal capacity. International *Journal of Law in Context*. 2014 Mar; 10(1):81-104.	Ireland	Examination of the regulation of personhood through the granting or denying of legal capacity	Discussion paper	Builds on work of Bach and Kerzner (2012), introducing 'enabling conditions' as having relevance. Suggests a newer approach as the 'support model' with different levels of support referred to as the 'continuum of support' envisaging 'enabling conditions' as ever-present accommodations which enable people to progress along the continuum of support
5)	Kohn NA, Blumenthal JA. A critical assessment of supported decision-making for persons aging with intellectual disabilities. *Disability and Health Journal.* 2014 Jan 31;7(1):S40-3.	United States of America	To review the evidence base for supported decision making (SDM) for aging persons with ID	Literature Review	SDM as a process by which a third party 'helps' an individual with ID. Of the reviewed literature findings are discursive identifying perceived benefits and challenges, a lack of evidence; substantial further research to explore effective evidence-based SDM practices to develop policy

Table 5. (Continued)

	Author(s) & Year & Journal	Country	Aim	Methodology and Design	Main Findings
6)	García Iriarte E, O'Brien P, Chadwick D. Involving people with intellectual disabilities within research teams: lessons learned from an Irish experience. *Journal of Policy and Practice in Intellectual Disabilities*. 2014 Jun 1;11(2):149-57.	Ireland	To review inclusive approaches to research	A reflective analysis	Paper describes main findings from three studies, focus groups with people with ID and supporters who conducted the research and interviews with people to whom the findings were disseminated The analysis suggested that a team approach including active supporters and experienced researchers was critical to their feasibility. How people with complex support needs, including those with profound and multiple disabilities can be involved in research endeavours has yet to be considered. Need for critical focus for ongoing investigation and reflection in this area.
7)	Lashewicz B, Mitchell J, Salami E, Cheuk S. Understanding and addressing voices of adults with disabilities within their family caregiving contexts:	Canada	A paper commissioned by the Law Commission Ontario, to provide background research for its Legal Capacity, Decision-Making	Narrative approach, Semi-structured interviews, funded by Canadian Institute for Health Research and	20 members from seven families all of which include and adult with a developmental disability (of various abilities) were interviewed, independently and together, 'detailed evidence of family

	Author(s) & Year & Journal	Country	Aim	Methodology and Design	Main Findings
	Implications for capacity, decision-making and guardianship. Toronto, Canada: Law Commission of Ontario.		and Guardianship project	conducted in Alberta between 2010 and 2012	caregivers facilitating equal footing by acting as respectful, supportive voices for their child or sibling with the use of prompting and clarifying questions that are effective yet not overbearing'
8)	Walker EM, Crawford F, Leonard H. Community participation: Conversations with parent-carers of young women with Rett syndrome. *Journal of Intellectual and Developmental Disability*. 2014 Jul 3;39(3).243-52.	Australia	Exploration of challenges that people with PIMD face to participating in their community	Qualitative interpretive approach Sample; parent carers of nine carers from six families	Majority of parents recalled positive social connections saw social participation as unrealistic expectation related to communication impairments of daughters.
9)	Carney T. Participation and service access rights for people with intellectual disability: A role for law?. *Journal of Intellectual and Developmental Disability*. 2013 Mar 1;38(1):59-69.	Australia	Discusses legislations role in supporting personal autonomy	Exploratory discursive paper, classified under 'Opinions and Perspectives'	SDM and personal budgets for services are the new paradigms and this paper explores the part to be played by law in achieving social justice objectives of securing rights to human services or health care; a major challenge in any sphere.
10	Chadwick DD, Mannan H, Garcia Iriarte E, McConkey R, O'brien P, Finlay F, Lawlor A,	Ireland	The aim of this study was to map life experiences of families with an ID member whilst involving some	Participatory action research a mixed method approach;	Few studies in Ireland that address family life for this cohort, research was funded by a Marie Curie Transfer of

Table 5. (Continued)

	Author(s) & Year & Journal	Country	Aim	Methodology and Design	Main Findings
	Harrington G. Family voices: life for family carers of people with intellectual disabilities in Ireland. *Journal of Applied Research in Intellectual Disabilities*. 2013 Mar 1;26(2):119-32.		family members as co-researchers	focus groups and online survey	Knowledge Fellowship to the National Institute for Intellectual Disability TCD. Decided to include this article as it describes family life for families. not feeling included, involved and consulted. where decisions had been made without their 'input'
11	Clarke G, Harrison K, Holland A, Kuhn I, Barclay S. How are treatment decisions made about artificial nutrition for individuals at risk of lacking capacity? A systematic literature review. *PLoS One*. 2013 Apr 16;8(4):e61475.	United Kingdom	To review and synthesis the international evidence on treatment decisions concerning artificial	Literature Review, 66 papers included 49 involved people with dementia, 30 people with acquired brain injuries (ABI), and four people with ID	There are ethically complex decisions surrounding tube feeding with quality of life the main decision-making factor but its meaning varied; prolonging life was the second most cited factor; patient's wishes were influential but not determinative; families had some influence but were infrequently involved in final recommendations. Four studies were identified relating to ID revealing a lack of research in this patient group.
12	Doyle S, Flynn E. Ireland's ratification of the UN convention on the rights of persons	Ireland	Overview of the current situation in Ireland in relation to	Discursive paper	'Stumbling block' in Irish law Lunacy Regulation (Ireland) Act 1871 is outlined as it presents with

	Author(s) & Year & Journal	Country	Aim	Methodology and Design	Main Findings
	with disabilities: challenges and opportunities. British *Journal of Learning Disabilities*. 2013 Sep 1;41(3):171-80.		ratification of the UN- CRPD.		challenges to the ratification of the UN-CRPD. Requirements of Article 12 are outlined, as is the prelude to the Assisted Decision Making Bill (2013) presented.
13	Gooding P. Supported decision-making: a rights-based disability concept and its implications for mental health law. *Psychiatry, Psychology and Law*. 2013 Jun 1;20(3):431-51.	Australia	To clarify the concept of SDM and to consider its major implications for *mental health law*	Discursive paper	Describes the intersection of international and national law, policy and programming whose success 'can only truly be measured 'on the ground' for those whose lives' it is meant to assist. A comprehensive and insightful review of legislation and emerging examples of SDM practices are reviewed.
14	McConkey R, Bunting B, Ferry F, Iriarte EG, Stevens R. An evaluation of personalised supports to individuals with disabilities and mental health difficulties.	Ireland	Evaluation of people's experiences moving from congregated settings to more personalised arrangements	Qualitative Interviews and focus groups	A Genio funded evaluation describing benefits of personalisation agenda from client, family and staff perspective. Overall more positive and cost neutral.
15	Kohn NA, Blumenthal JA, Campbell AT. Supported decision-making: A viable alternative to guardianship.	United States of America	To present an overarching review of concept, research, quality related issues and implementing concerns.	Review, non-systematic	Normative appeal of SDM, however little is known about how SDM processes operate or about the outcome of the processes.

Table 5. (Continued)

	Author(s) & Year & Journal	Country	Aim	Methodology and Design	Main Findings
	Penn St. L. Rev. 2012;117:1111.				Evidence to know the extent to it can remedy the problems posed by surrogate decision-making processes is not evident. Concerns with the potential to disempower people, specific research agendas to develop evidence base and guide future policy.
16	Werner S. Individuals with intellectual disabilities: a review of the literature on decision-making since the Convention on the Rights of People with Disabilities (CRPD). *Public Health Reviews.* 2012 Dec 2;34(2):14.	Israel	Map current decision making situations four years after the enactment of the CRPD to provide a base for comparison in future years	Systematic literature review on decision making among individuals with ID since the CRPD. 27 manuscripts reviewed	Examples of decision making approaches in adult transitioning, sexuality health care employment and self-advocacy reported from various countries. Recommendations of most studies identify improvements in supported decision making no comprehensive working model that was used and reviewed 'a task at hand for the future'.
17	Devi N, Bickenbach J, Stucki G. Moving towards substituted or supported decision-making? Article 12 of the Convention on the Rights of Persons with Disabilities.	USA	Makes the argument that interpretation of Article 12 of UN CRPD requires a SDM model to implement based on the history and the deliberation process of the CRPD	Discursive paper	Since the Convention entered into force in 2006, the literature on the concept of SDM is small but rapidly growing. Discusses a model of decision making by Bach and Kerzner (2010).

	Author(s) & Year & Journal	Country	Aim	Methodology and Design	Main Findings
	ALTER-European *Journal of Disability Research/Revue Européenne de Recherche sur le Handicap*. 2011 Dec 31;5(4):249-64.				Their model is intended to move away from assessing the mental capacity (decision-making ability) of a person, and look at facilitated and supported processes of ensuring liberty and autonomy
18	Dunn MC, Clare IC, Holland AJ. Living 'a life like ours' : support workers' accounts of substitute decision-making in residential care homes for adults with intellectual disabilities. *Journal of Intellectual Disability Research*. 2010 Feb 1;54(2):144-60.	United Kingdom	To build upon and develop recent empirical and ethical analyses of substitute decision-making in non-medical settings	Interviews and observations underpinning constructivist grounded theory study design	The value of adopting established principles and procedures for substitute decision-making in practice is uncertain. Support workers interpret substitute decision-making within a broad moral account of their care role, orientating their support towards 'helping residents to live "a life like ours" ', emerging as having explanatory power drawing on their own values and life experiences to shape the substitute decisions that they make on behalf of residents.
19	Bach M, Kerzner L. A new paradigm for protecting autonomy and the right to legal capacity Toronto: Law Commission of Ontario.	Canada	Commissioned paper by Law Commission of Ontario to provide background research for its Advancing Substantive Equality for	Discursive paper	The authors assert that the principles set out in the UN CRPD require a paradigm shift in the law of capacity so that the question is no longer: Does a person have the mental capacity to

Table 5. (Continued)

	Author(s) & Year & Journal	Country	Aim	Methodology and Design	Main Findings
			Persons with Disabilities through Law, Policy and Practice project		exercise legal capacity? The question is instead: What types of supports are required for the person to exercise his or her legal capacity? Question of 'meaningful' arises as is the recognition of 'shared life experiences and personal knowledge' philosophical, ethical and a mine field for the non-legal
20	Burton-Smith R, McVilly KR, Yazbeck M, Parmenter TR, Tsutsui T. Service and support needs of Australian carers supporting a family member with disability at home. *Journal of intellectual and developmental disability*. 2009 Sep 1;34(3):239-47.	Australia	To examine variables that are central to the principle of Nirje's (1973) normalisation principles and their influence on choice availability for people with and without ID	Quantitative, survey n=448 parents and carers	Level of disability rather than age affected opportunities for choice making with choice availability significantly lower for adults with more severe degrees of disability than for people with milder intellectual disability. Thus, in the realm of' daily choice' normalisation appears to be problematic for individuals who have moderate or greater degrees of intellectual disability.

	Author(s) & Year & Journal	Country	Aim	Methodology and Design	Main Findings
21	Neely-Barnes S, Carolyn Graff J, Marcenko M, Weber L. Family decision making: Benefits to persons with developmental disabilities and their family members. *Intellectual and Developmental Disabilities*. 2008 Apr;46(2):93-105.	United States of America (only data from Washington state used)	Three hypothesis related to different patterns of family involvement in decision making about services	Quantitative, Survey design Sample; =547, Family carers, randomly selected, Data were analyzed using SPSS 13.0 (SPSS, 2004) and Mplus version 3.1	Family involvement in planning and choosing services has become a key intervention concept in developmental disability services. Identified 4 cohorts 1) involved in decision making (n = 118), 2) involved only in planning (n =166), involved only in financial decisions (n =75), and uninvolved (n =188).4.8% respondents identified that the persons they were caring for had a profound intellectual disability, the lowest % of all categories. The more involvement indicated more satisfaction with services and more family satisfaction.
22	Hogg J. Complex needs and complex solutions: the challenge of profound intellectual and multiple disabilities. *Journal of Policy and Practice in Intellectual Disabilities*. 2007 Jun 1;4(2):79-82.	Scotland	Identifies key issues affecting people with PIMD	Discursive paper	Philosophical paper, comparing the eugenic and bioethicists schools beliefs of how persons with PIMD have no self-awareness and therefore cannot self-determine; attributes which define personhood and thus the concept of nonperson exists implementation of social, educational, and health policies placing people with

Table 5. (Continued)

	Author(s) & Year & Journal	Country	Aim	Methodology and Design	Main Findings
23					PIMD within a framework that facilitates the realisation of individual aspirations and enhances their personal
24	Petry K, Maes B. Description of the support needs of people with profound multiple disabilities using the 2002 AAMR system: An overview of literature. *Education and Training in developmental Disabilities*. 2007 Jun 1:130-43.	United States of America	Describes support needs of people with profound multiple disabilities (PMD),	Discussion paper based on study of the literature	Theoretical model of disability presented, where the functioning of people with ID can be understood from the interaction of factors on five dimensions. The concept 'interaction' implies that these dimensions are not independent. Based on the five basic dimensions of the 2002 AAMR System, being intellectual abilities, adaptive behaviour, participation, interaction and social roles, health and context
25	Turnbull A, Turnbull R. Self-determination for individuals with significant cognitive disabilities and their families. *Journal of the Association for Persons with Severe Handicaps*.	United States of America	Discusses the role of families in supporting the self-determination of individuals with significant cognitive disabilities	Personal, Discursive paper by two parents (allied to healthcare professionals)	Research should be based on the "wisdom of the grassroots' to conceptualise and operationalise self-determination from the perspectives of individuals with significant cognitive disabilities and their families.

	Author(s) & Year & Journal	Country	Aim	Methodology and Design	Main Findings
	2001 Mar;26(1):56-62.				This paper demonstrates the reality and complexity of supporting self-determination development for an individual with an intellectual disability and the role of (or lack of) the state, service providers that honour family and individual culture.
26	Gordon RM. The emergence of assisted (supported) decision-making in the Canadian law of adult guardianship and substitute decision-making. International *Journal of Law and Psychiatry*. 2000 Feb 29;23(1):61-77.	Canada	To contextualise the transition from guardianship approach to assisted decision making approaches	Discursive paper	Argues that independent decision-making is a myth; that every adult uses interdependent decision-making in the course of getting through the day. Assisted decision-making has set the impetus for reconsiderations of taken-for-granted concepts: the common law presumption of capability and the sanctity of independent decision-making.

Appraising and synthesising the literature

There are different ways of appraising and synthesising the literature and the format by Wright et al. (31) supports the notion of 'building a picture' involves identifying the main themes or ideas on the subject that commonly occur in the literature. Identifying these areas requires making links between the points being raised in the literature and formulating new ideas about aspects of the subject (31), in that regard, the literature review is structured hereafter.

REVIEW FINDINGS

The literature review had an aim; to identify what is known about 'how family carers' support persons with a PIMD in decision making?' And secondly 'Considerations when involving people with profound intellectual and multiple disability in decision-making'. Review findings are presented in three sections; 1) General information and background 2) models of SDM and 3) challenges within a "principle based concept."

General information and background of SDM

In relation to the review questions a disappointing outcome found no evidence to depict how family carers' experienced supporting persons, living with PIMD, in decision-making, the majority of papers reflected paid workers. The review therefore broadened original scope to included policy and grey literature and that of other supporters of persons, living with PIMD.

It is clearly evident from the literature review SDM is emerging as a fast growing liberator in the disabilities domain. This is partly due to the influence of the CRPD and advances in practice which advocate for replacement of paternalistic/patriarchal substitute decision-making by the autonomous and dignity enhancing concept that SDM purports to be. Since 2006, a rise in papers exploring the concept, construct and approaches to SDM has arisen partly due to the implementation of the CRPD. Ireland, Australia, Canada, United States of America and the United Kingdom are countries in which the discussion papers mainly derived from.

Agreement related to the concept of SDM 'as an ideal principle' evident throughout all policies and papers reviewed, yet the theoretical papers were more focused in their criticisms of SDM identifying it as problematic (32), undefined and challenging (33) as complicated aspects as the process evolve (19, 20). With the 'wing in its sails' (32) conceptually SDM has been described as ideal yet enigmatic and ill-defined requiring more substantial theory of practice (34). Part of this ambiguity relates to the lack of a clear or agreed definition of SDM (35), and this has proven to be problematic and a contributory factor towards confusion and ambiguity (15).

Examination of the policies and literature provides an understanding of how difficult it is to make such a seemingly simple normative concept applied. Clear evidence from this examination demonstrates:

- A will and drive to support individuals with disabilities to engage in making real and every day choices in their lives is clearly evident. Interventions to support these policies tended to be less available, descriptive and primarily from a healthcare perspective as opposed to family carers
- The 'personal outcomes' approach is very evident in policies reviewed aiming to ensure services are provided in an optimum manner and in a way which is responsive to the wishes of service users and their families. A key challenge will lie in balancing the emphasis on autonomy with principles of beneficence, mutuality and care
- A significant shift in 'best interests' to 'will and preferences' is noted. More research is needed to understand how best to ascertain the will and preferences of an individual with significant communicative or cognitive challenges
- A rights-based approach to service provision and equality of access to services; access to services and supports; choice by persons and maximising individual potential is presented to aspire to the values of maintain dignity and respect for all, ensuring good and ordinary living and aspirations of all people are realised

From an Irish perspective, a significant development in Irish capacity legislation was the introduction of the Assisted Decision Making (Capacity) Act (2015) which will have substantial implications for persons, living with PIMD, their families and professionals who support. The Act reforms Ireland's Capacity legislation which has been in place since the 1870s by establishing a modern statutory framework to support decision-making by adults who have difficulty in making decisions without help. It will repeal the Marriage of Lunatics Act 1811 and the Lunacy Regulation (Ireland) Act 1871. Within the act is the understanding that legal capacity assessment changes from the current "all or nothing status" approach to a "flexible functional definition" whereby capacity is assessed only in relation to the matter in question and only at the time in question. If a person is found to lack decision-making capacity in one matter, this will not necessarily mean that s/he also lacks capacity in another matter. The Act recognises that capacity can fluctuate in certain cases.

Recognising the fluctuating nature of capacity, "Decision-Making Support Options" are to be made available. The Act proposes three types of decision-making support options to respond to the range of support needs that people may have in relation to decision-making capacity. With each of the three decision-making support options decisions can be made on personal welfare, property and finance or a combination of both. These supports are classified as:

- Assisted decision-making: a person may appoint a decision-making assistant – typically a family member or carer – through a formal decision-making assistance agreement to support him or her to access information or to understand, make and express decisions. Decision-making responsibility remains with the person. The decision-making assistant will be supervised by the Director of the Decision Support Service.
- Co-decision-making: a person can appoint a trusted family member or friend as a co-decision-maker to make decisions jointly with him or her under a co-decision-making agreement. Decision-making responsibility is shared jointly between the person and the

co-decision-maker. The co-decision-maker will be supervised by the Director of the Decision Support Service.

- Decision-making representative: for the small minority of people who are not able to make decisions even with help, the Act provides for the Circuit Court to appoint a decision-making representative. A decision-making representative will make decisions on behalf of the person but must abide by the guiding principles and must reflect the person's will and preferences where possible. The functions of decision-making representatives will be as limited in scope and duration as is reasonably practicable (Assisted Decision Making (Capacity) Act 2015).

The provisions of the Act will be commenced on a phased basis to coincide with the ratification of the UN Convention of the Rights of Persons with Disabilities anticipated in 2017. Therefore in comparison to our UK, USA and other European counterparts we have much to advance in the area of SDM, but our framework in the legal context appears to marry that of existing models in the literature now outlined.

Models of supporting decision making

Two SDM models were found within the literature reviewed; Back and Kerzner (15) 'Maximising decision making abilities' and Flynn and Arstein-Kerslake (20) 'Enabling conditions' who built on the work of the Back and Kerzner. Back and Kerzner conceptualise SDM as a mechanism for enhancing a person's ability to make his/her own decisions, thus, an apparently "incapable person" may be able to make his/her own decisions with the help of others, and thus exercise his/her own legal capacity. Supports may function to do the following:

- assist in formulating one's purposes, to explore the range of choices and to make a decision

- engage in the decision-making process with other parties to make agreements that give effect to one's decision, where one's decisions requires this

Bach and Kerzner view of SDM as a process with outcomes views SDM as:

> occurring when an individual with cognitive challenges is the ultimate decision-maker but is provided support from one or more persons who explain issues to the individual and, where necessary, interpret the individual's words and behaviour to determine his or her preferences through three different decision-making statuses.

1) Legally independent status - has the ability, by him or herself or with assistance, to understand and appreciate the information relevant to, and the reasonably foreseeable consequences of, making a decision
2) Supported decision-making status - a support person is appointed by the person with a disability, or by an administrative tribunal or court. Due to a relationship with the person with a disability, the support person can interpret and carry out his or her will or intention, "consistent with the person's identity" and respecting "the individual's dignity of risk." The support person would be obligated to consult with the person he or she is supporting and to make decisions based on that consultation.
3) Facilitated decision-making status- a facilitator is appointed by administrative tribunal or advanced planning document (i.e., power of attorney). Facilitated status would not "represent a statement or judgment about their cognitive status or abilities," simply that they do not meet the criteria, above, of legal independence, and do not have anyone in their life who know them well enough to interpret their will and/or intention (15).

The conceptualisation of SDM purported by Bach and Kerzner as a process with outcomes has underpinnings in decision-making capability is seen as a relationship between decision-making abilities, decision-making supports and accommodations, and decision-making status. People move between statuses as abilities, supports and accommodations evolve reflected in their image below;

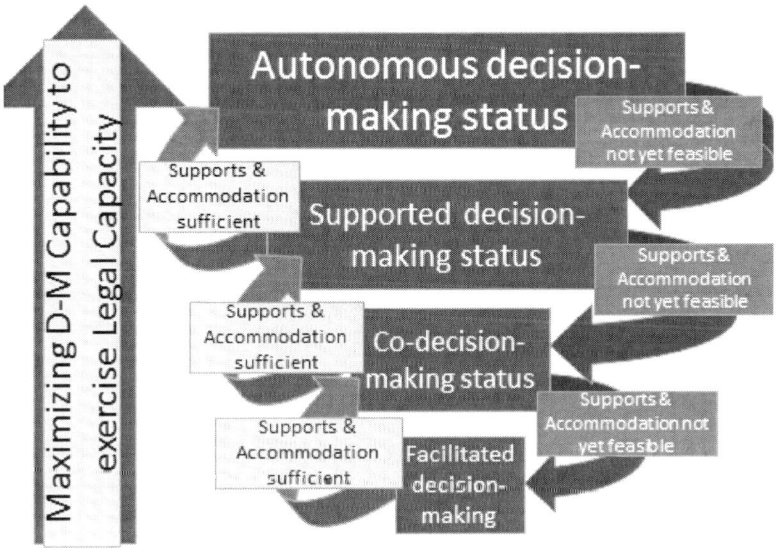

Figure 1. Bach and Kerzner (2010) SDM 'maximizing decision making capacity'.

This approach to 'decision making capacity' while focusing on what accommodations and supports a person requires to manage the decision-making process in a way that maximizes their decision making capacity, and thus exercise legal capacity, given their unique decision-making abilities has the potential to fall in to the trap of 'capacity assessment' which ultimately is a challenge to Article 12 of the UN- CRPD. Acknowledging that Back and Kerzner did not intend that this model be used to determine whether or not a person has legal capacity, but rather the status through which legal capacity is exercised in particular when disputes arise in this regard among parties in a decision-making process. Building on the work of Back and Kerzner, Flynn and Arstein-Kerslake (2014) purpose the 'support model' to SDM presented in the image below.

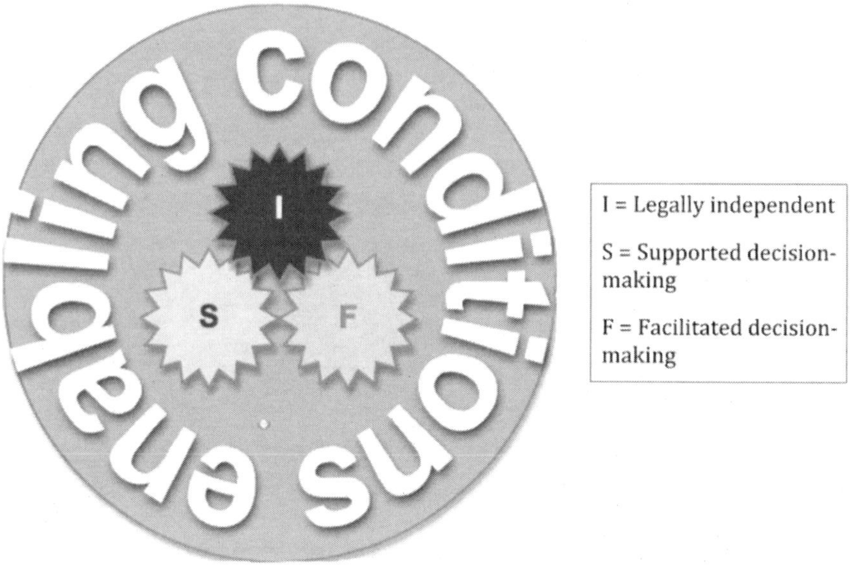
enabling conditions
I
S
F
I = Legally independent
S = Supported decision-making
F = Facilitated decision-making

Figure 2. Flynn and Arstein-Kerslake (2014) SDM 'support model'.

The first principle in this model is that every person enjoys legal capacity regardless of her level of decision-making ability, and should be empowered to exercise her legal capacity through the expression of her will and preference. Second, this requires the abolition of any assessment of decision-making ability which may results in the loss of legal capacity. Any assessment which takes place in a support model of legal capacity should be centred on the support that is needed in decision-making to augment an individual's existing strengths, rather than the deficits of the individual. Finally, the support model requires the abolition of substitute decision-making which subjects the will of an individual to the dominance of another's will or notion of what is in her 'best interest'.

This does not prevent a representative from making a decision for another person who is not expressing her will and preferences in a way which anyone can interpret – rather, it requires representatives making such decisions to do so in a way which attempts to draw out the imagined will and preferences of the person (20). Flynn and Arstein-Kerslake 'support model' image represents the overarching support model of legal capacity. The cogs in the centre of the circle represent the three clusters of decision-making as described by Bach and Kerzner: legally independent, supported and facilitated. Surrounding these clusters and captured within the overarching support model are the enabling conditions – which include advocacy, reasonable accommodation, accessible information and communication, recognition of different forms of expression, advance planning tools, and so on.

It is important to note that Flynn and Arstein-Kerslake model is intended to demonstrate that the presence of the enabling conditions may move someone from one cluster of decision-making to another – for example, from supported decision-making to legally independent decision-making. Conversely, the absence of the enabling conditions might lead to an individual requiring more intensive forms of support in decision-making, such as a facilitated decision-maker. Even where the enabling conditions are present, external factors, such as the person's environment, might result in the person remaining in the same decision-making cluster for most of their adult life. However, this does not diminish the purpose of the enabling conditions or reduce the obligation to ensure that they are in place.

Challenges that may arise with this model are identification and remuneration for the role of the "representatives making such decisions to do so in a way which attempts to draw out the imagined will and preferences of the person." Family carers have traditionally provided the majority of support and assistance for persons, living with PIMD, for example where to live, what clothes to wear, leisure and employment activities, and support to engage in health educational and social activities such as going to the dentist, doctor and school. Are we to assume that family carers should continue this role and are therefore bound by this new approach to support or will appointees be allocated as supporter, perhaps against family wishes?

A second challenge to this model is understanding of the term 'the imagined will and preferences'. The unintentional nature of communication associated with persons, living with PIMD, is well noted as is the problematic nature of communicating intentions. We need to question if the representation of 'the imagined will of another' promotes self-determination or promotes the supporters understanding of another's identity and intended choice making. The subtle difference between these two points is crucial to the purpose of the model itself, and the danger of camouflaging the person, living with PIMD, identity and choice making assertions may be lost in the supporter asserting an 'imagined will and preferences': in the absence of corroboration or confirmation. A suggestion to replace 'imagined' with 'attempt to assert the person's will and preferences' may be beneficial to the model being implemented and more realistic to the challenges that people face in this endeavour.

To summarise both models, Back and Kerzner and Flynn and Arstein-Kerslake are reflective of changing times. The assumptions that all persons can make decisions are implicit and explicit in their discussions. Ethical, legal and practical challenges of understanding and implementing such models of support require further understanding and research.

Challenges within a "principle based concept"

The third finding of the literature review 'Challenges within a principle based concept' reflects the call for movement beyond rhetoric towards action and empirical evidence directly evaluating SDM. The literature reviewed described the conceptual basis of SDM from an epistemological and linguistic perspective. Supporting decision making as purported by the UN CRPD refers to 'those assisting a person may communicate the individual's intentions to others or help him/her understand the choices at hand. They may help others to realize that a person with significant disabilities is also a person with a history, interest and aims in life, and is someone capable of exercising his/her legal capacity' formed on the basis of human values and focused on the unique needs of the disabled person (epistemological principle). There is consistency in the meaning of the

SDM as a central value of the supporter-supported interaction (linguistic principle) evident throughout the reviewed literature.

The necessity of the conceptual clarity addresses the many reflections and philosophical debates in the literature reviewed of the 'hard cases' and the question 'do persons, living with PIMD have self-awareness and can they self-determine'. Discourses of historical eugenic programmes, derogatory and inhuman institutional practices in the name of 'care' with dismissive and negative attitudes to those with severe impairments was presented. The principled nature of SDM therefore is warranted. Moving forward, operational understandings is required. While understanding that SDM approaches require all people be known as masters of their own lives, with a life plan, pathway, a life story or narrative education, training and further research are warranted to address the fundamental aspect to deliver the aspiration of SDM.

In this vein, it is worrying how SDM was presented in the literature as a 'wonder drug'. This wonder drug was presented as counteracting the paternalistic and infantilising approaches that hinder individual aspirations and personal development that disabled people have reported. Theoretical papers over policy documents were critical of the concept 'SDM' in that overcoming challenges related to realising equality, support, and protection, central for people, living with PIMD, are limited by legislation in its own right. Overcoming challenges in discrimination, inequality and poor resources has financial, attitudinal and social infrastructure requirements. This is important to acknowledge, as it can be misleading to individuals living with PIMD and their supporters to think 'it's all fixed now that we recognise your capacity'.

People, living with PIMD, require full time care and support in all activities of living, this is the nature of their impairments. Supporters play an important role to interpret their communication intent. These are well accepted aspects of providing support to this group of people. Providing persons, living with PIMD, opportunities to exercise their legal capacity and demonstrate self-determination connects to the principles of therapeutic or effective communication requiring attention to multiple, interacting factors. Carney (32) recommendations are helpful in this regard and worth noting:

- effective communication, including the provision of information and advice to a person and through ensuring that a person is able to communicate their decisions to others
- spending time to determine a person' s preferences and wishes
- informal relationships of support between a person and members of their social networks
- agreements or appointments to indicate that a relationship of support exists; statutory relationships of support— whether through private or court/tribunal appointment

Support by its nature, is to offer resources and by doing so influence the lives and wellbeing of people, living with PIMD, arguably their survival and being lies in external support and influence. Approaches to SDM now require pragmatic principles addressing the process, functions and outcomes in real terms for those experiencing supporting and supported.

Summary of contributions within the literature review

The review has highlighted that as of 2006, this generation of people with disabilities is the first generation with the rights and opportunities protected and promoted by the UN CRPD. Secondly, the time to move SDM from theory to practice is now upon us. There is clear evidence of the need for more explicit research informed by evidence as to the processes of SDM, implementation and evaluation of such processes to inform future policy.

Agreement in the literature and policies is that people require a range of supports to make decisions in their lives. Turning their decision-making abilities into decision-making capabilities a significant finding of this literature review is the lack of research relevant to family carers supporting persons, living with PIMD, in decision making.

Strengths and limitations of the review

The strength of this literature review relates to the variation in papers reviewed, in conjunction with discussion and policy perspectives which yielded broad and overarching findings that assisted in exploring how family carers support persons, living with disabilities, in decision making. This review may have missed salient recent findings, negative findings, and other reports by non-profit organizations. Findings are mostly comprised of Western ideologies and provisions. This may be due to the search strategy, which was limited to articles published in English. Perhaps including non-published studies and studies published in languages other than English may affect the findings of this review.

CONCLUSION

The literature review aimed to explore the empirical literature to ascertain family carers' experiences of supporting persons, living with PIMD, in decision making. This literature review diverted from a systematic to an eclectic approach due to the absence of literature pertaining to families' carers' experiences supporting persons, living with PIMD, in decision making.

Findings from the review reflects the change in policy and law with regard to legal capacity. Academic literature and governmental polices elicit the background, models and challenges to implementing a seemingly normative concept, SDM. The obligation to 'support' means that in cases such as supporting persons, living with PIMD, efforts have to be made to augment existing capacity and grow capabilities to realise the vision of Article 12. Producing research that informs this obligation in pragmatic terms is clearly upon us.

REFERENCES

[1] Department of Justice Equality and Law Reform. National Disability strategy, Dublin: Department of Justice Equality Law Reform, 2004.

[2] United Nations Convention on the rights of persons with disabilities. Optional protocol to the Convention 2006. New York: United Nations General Assembly, 2006.

[3] Department of Health, Valuing People Now; A new three-year strategy for people with learning disabilities, London: Stationery Office, 2009.

[4] Health Service Executive, Time to move on from Congregated Settings: a strategy for community inclusion-Report of the working group on congregated settings, Dublin: Health Service Executive, 2011.

[5] Chadwick DD, Mannan H, Garcia Iriarte E, McConkey R, O'Brien P, Finlay F, et al. Family voices: life for family carers of people with intellectual disabilities in Ireland, J Appl Res Intellect Disabil 2013:26(2):119-32.

[6] Twigg J, Atkin K. Carers perceived: policy and practice in informal care. London: McGraw-Hill Education UK, 1994.

[7] Heaton J. The gaze and visibility of the carer: a Foucauldian analysis of the discourse of informal care. Sociol Health Illness 1999;21(6):759-77.

[8] Cummins RA. The subjective well-being of people caring for a family member with a severe disability at home: A review. J Intellect Dev Disabil 2001;26(1):83-100.

[9] Burton-Smith R, McVilly KR, Yazbeck M, Parmenter TR, Tsutsui T. Service and support needs of Australian carers supporting a family member with disability at home. J Intellect Dev Disabil 2009;34(3):239-47.

[10] Department of Health. The national carers strategy: Recognised, supported, empowered. Dublin: Department Health, 2012.

[11] Coyle CE, Kramer J, Mutchler JE. Aging together: Sibling carers of adults with intellectual and developmental disabilities. J Policy Pract Intellect Disabil 2014;11(4):302-12.

[12] Kavanaugh MS, Noh H, Studer L. "It'd be nice if someone asked me how I was doing. Like,'cause I will have an answer": exploring support needs of young carers of a parent with Huntington's disease. Vulnerable Child Youth Stud 2015;10(1):12-25.

[13] Lunsky Y, Tint A, Robinson S, Gordeyko M, Ouellette-Kuntz H. System-wide information about family carers of adults with intellectual/developmental disabilities: A scoping review of the literature. J Policy Pract Intellect Disabil 2014;11(1):8-18.

[14] McPherson KM, Kayes NK, Moloczij N, Cummins C. Improving the interface between informal carers and formal health and social services: a qualitative study. Int J Nurs Stud 2014;51(3):418-29.

[15] Bach M, Kerzner L. A new paradigm for protecting autonomy and the right to legal capacity. Toronto, ON: Law Commission of Ontario, 2010.
[16] Devi N, Bickenbach J, Stucki G. Moving towards substituted or supported decision-making? Article 12 of the Convention on the Rights of Persons with Disabilities. ALTER-Eur J Disabil Res 2011;5(4):249-64.
[17] Schalock RL, Borthwick-Duffy SA, Bradley VJ, Buntinx WH, Coulter DL, Craig EM, et al. Intellectual disability: Definition, classification, and systems of supports. Washington, DC: American Association Intellectual and Developmental Disabilities, 2010.
[18] McConkey R, Bunting B, Ferry F, Iriarte EG, Stevens R. An evaluation of personalised supports to individuals with disabilities and mental health difficulties. Mullingar: Genio Trust, 2013.
[19] Flynn E, Arstein-Kerslake A. Legislating personhood: Realising the right to support in exercising legal capacity. Int J Law Context 2014; 10(1):81-104.
[20] Flynn E, Arstein-Kerslake A. The support model of legal capacity: Fact, fiction, or fantasy? Berkeley J Int Law (BJIL) 2014;32(1):4.
[21] Tadema AC, Vlaskamp C. The time and effort in taking care for children with profound intellectual and multiple disabilities: A study on care load and support. Br J Learn Disabil 2010;38(1):41-8.
[22] Kelly C. Making 'care' accessible: Personal assistance for disabled people and the politics of language. Crit Soc Policy 2011:31(4):562-82.
[23] Moran N, Arksey H, Glendinning C, Jones K, Netten A, Rabiee P. Personalisation and carers: Whose rights? Whose benefits? Br J Soc Work 2011;42(3):461-79.
[24] Department of the Environment, Community and Local Government. National housing strategy for people with a disability 2011- 016, Dublin: Environment Community Local Government, 2011.
[25] James N. The formal support experiences of family carers of people with an intellectual disability who also display challenging behaviour and/or mental health issues: What do carers say? J Intellect Disabil 2013;17(1):6-23.
[26] Power A. 'It's the system working for the system': Carers' experiences of learning disability services in Ireland. Health Soc Care Commun 2009;17(1):92-8.
[27] Moher D, Liberati A, Tetzlaff J, Altman DG. Preferred reporting items for systematic reviews and meta-analyses: the PRISMA statement. Ann Int Med 2009;151:264-9.
[28] Clarke G, Harrison K, Holland A, Kuhn I, Barclay S. How are treatment decisions made about artificial nutrition for individuals at risk of lacking capacity? A systematic literature review. PLoS One 2013;8(4):e61475.
[29] Bellamy G, Croot L, Bush A, Berry H, Smith A. A study to define: profound and multiple learning disabilities (PMLD). J Intellec Disabil 2010;14(3):221-35.
[30] Wallace M, Wray A. Critical reading and writing for postgraduates, 2nd ed. London: Sage, 2011.

[31] Wright K, Street P, Gousy M. Academic skills: using literature to support your discussion. Br J Nurs 2011;20(2):102-6.

[32] Carney T. Clarifying, operationalising, and evaluating supported decision making models. Res Pract Intellect Dev Disabil 2014;1(1):46-50.

[33] Werner S. Individuals with intellectual disabilities: a review of the literature on decision-making since the Convention on the Rights of People with Disabilities (CRPD). Public Health Rev 2012;34(2):14.

[34] Browning M, Bigby C, Douglas J. Supported decision making: Understanding how its conceptual link to legal capacity is influencing the development of practice. Res Pract Intellect Dev Disabil 2014;1(1):34-45.

[35] Kohn NA, Blumenthal JA, Campbell AT. Supported decision-making: A viable alternative to guardianship. Penn St Law Rev 2012;117:1111.

In: Intellectual Disability
Editors: Ariel Tenenbaum et al.
ISBN: 978-1-53617-866-1

Chapter 7

LEARNING, MOTOR AND MENTAL HEALTH PROFILES IN PUPILS WITH BORDERLINE INTELLECTUAL FUNCTIONING AND AVERAGE INTELLECTUAL FUNCTIONING

Marianna Alesi**, PhD and Gaetano Rappo, PhD
Department of di Psychological, Pedagogical and Educational Sciences,
University of Palermo, Italy

ABSTRACT

There is a lack of research addressing the study of the borderline intellectual functioning (BIF) in school-aged population. In children and adolescents with BIF high rates of school complaints, movement impairments and mental health disorders have been demonstrated. In children and adolescents with BIF high rates of school complaints, movement impairments and mental health disorders have been demonstrated. This study aims at comparing learning, motor and mental

* Corresponding Author: Marianna Alesi, Associate professor, Dipartimento di Scienze Psicologiche, Pedagogiche e della Formazione, University of Palermo, V le delle Scienze, Edificio 15, 90128 Palermo, Italy. E-mail: marianna.alesi@unipa.it.

health profiles showed by pupils with BIF and pupils with average intellectual functioning (AIF). Participants were 19 children with BIF and 19 with AIF. Learning, motor and mental health profiles were measured by multiple tests. Results show that pupils with BIF showed lower comprehension and decoding reading abilities, lower word and non word reading as well as lower mathematical abilities. Moreover impaired locomotion and object control skills and lower quotient of gross-motor ability were found in this group. BIF pupils showed lower self-esteem and higher rates of anxiety and depressed mood than typically developing children. On the whole, these findings document the high risk of co-occurrence among BIF, poor school performance, motor diseases and mental health impairment. Multifaceted educational and clinical interventions are needed to reduce or limit the risk of comorbidity in this population from school-age as well as to prevent negative evolution and improve cognitive and social functioning.

INTRODUCTION

Borderline intellectual functioning (BIF) is a heterogeneous lifelong condition generally identified as scoring between 1 and 2 standard deviations below the IQ mean (range 70-85) with a prevalence of 13.6% in the general population (1). However, despite its elevated occurrence, this intellectual condition is unrecognized and frequently misinterpreted, as pointed out by the large variety of verbal labels used as synonyms: subaverage intellectual functioning, borderline capacity, slow learning or backward learning (2, 3). In recent years research interest has grown, but insufficient studies have been developed till now. Peltopuro et al. (4) undertook a systematic literature review on the Borderline Intellectual Functioning and selected only 49 studies published till 2010 meeting inclusion criteria of IQ value ranging 70-84 IQ scores (4). The authors outlined an interesting geographical map being evidence for a wide gap between countries in scientific research addressing BIF. Limited to studies included in the above-mentioned review, 39% were carried out in the United States, 18% in the Netherlands, 12% in the United Kingdom, 8% in Germany, 6% in India, 4% in Australia, 0,02% in Italia, 0,02% in Norway, 0.02% in Finland, 0.02% in New Zealand, 0.02% in Sweden and 0.02% in

Iran. This leads authors to conclude that borderline intellectual functioning "is almost invisible in the field of research" (4). One possible explanation is the lack of an early and clear diagnostic model.

Ample evidence has been found associating BIF and poor scholastic performance in reading, writing or calculation areas as well as impaired abilities crucial to literacy such as memory, reasoning, attention and concentration and verbal fluency (5-8). An elevated frequency of comorbidity with poor school performance (89.1%), difficulties in writing (92.7%) and mathematics (76.4%) has been documented (9). In Italy, Vianello (10) postulated a rate of comorbidity between BIF and learning disabilities (LD) of about 1 each 408-571 pupils on the basis of the guidelines of Italian Consensus Conference (10). Specifically intellectual profiles of pupils with BIF and LD revealed a high discrepancy between the two global indexes obtained by the WISC-IV: GAI (general ability index) measuring the general intellectual abilities and CPI (cognitive proficiency index) measuring the processing skills. In detail, the GAI, derived by the subtests of verbal comprehension (VCI) and perceptual reasoning (PRI), was higher than the CPI derived by the subtests of working memory (WMI) and processing speed (PSI). Therefore, children with BIF and LD exhibited an intellectual profile characterized by better performance on verbal comprehension and perceptual reasoning and impaired abilities on working memory and processing speed. Furthermore in BIF pupils a characteristic profile of compromised verbal and visuo-spatial working memory and executive functions, such as inhibition skills and switch, has been evidenced (5, 11).

BIF pupils showed a specific weakness in the speed of information processing (SIP) by limiting the amount of information that can be processed in a given time interval (12-14). Abnormal cortical and subcortical gray matter (GM) volumes development was advanced to be responsible of this weakness (15). BIF pupils, compared to typically developing children (TDC) were found to have increased regional GM volume in bilateral sensorimotor and right posterior temporal cortex and decreased GM volume in the right parahippocampal gyrus associated with decrement in size in the right parahippocampal gyrus. Specifically, the first one is involved in visuo-motor abilities and visual control of skilled actions, whilst the parahippocampal gyrus and medial temporal lobe are involved in episodic memory development.

Recent research has addressed motor impairments in children with developmental disabilities showing delays in walking, deficits in fine motor skills, writing difficulties and low manual dexterity abilities (16, 17). To the best of our knowledge, only two studies have targeted the gross-motor development in BIF population (18, 19). BIF children, compared to TDC, poorly performed on a gross-motor development test as TGM (20, 21), one of the most frequently used tools to measure gross-motor development. In detail, BIF children underscored on the two subtests named locomotion (e.g., walking, running, hopping, galloping, jumping, sliding and leaping) and object-control tasks (e.g., throwing, catching, striking, bouncing, kicking, pulling and pushing). Object-control abilities appeared to be more impaired than locomotion ones. This is because of their higher cognitive load; the performance on tasks as throwing, catching and striking involves more sophisticated cognitive process linked to goal-directed behaviours or executive functions (18, 22). Whilst, locomotor tasks, such as walking, running and hopping, require stereotypic movements encompassing more automatized cognitive functioning. Consequently, locomotor skills didn't reveal differences among BIF children and peers with TD, but appeared to be more impaired when BIF pupils were compared to children with mild intellectual disability (18). Further evidence of interplay between intellectual and gross-motor abilities stems from exercise intervention programs. In their meta-analysis on benefits of motor programs in individuals with intellectual disabilities, Shin and Park (23) found out some general improvements following short-duration interventions (31-60 min.) and programs running 4 times per week (23). However, the efficacy of these programs was more consistent in younger individuals and with BIF. Recently Chen et al. (24) implemented a tennis table training over 16-weeks addressed to school-age children with borderline-to-mild intellectual functioning. Improvements on visual–perceptual abilities, abstract reasoning and shifting strategies were found in the BIF group compared to the control group (24).

Finally, a variety of studies demonstrated how BIF children are a high risk of mental health disorders population as increasing demands of contemporary society for superior levels of intellectual functioning enhance this risk for psychopathology since early childhood (25-27). It has been proved that a large number of children with BIF are more likely to have higher rates of anxiety and depression, develop neurotic and personality disorders (28, 29) and show higher levels of emotional impairments such as inadequate self-image, low self-esteem, poor self-concept with consequent interference with daily functioning (30-32). Pupils with BIF (mean age = 9.5 yrs.), compared to gifted intellectual functioning (GIF) and peers with average intellectual functioning (AIF), disclosed the lowest level of self-esteem and the highest levels of school anxiety and depression mood (31). Moreover, children with BIF are more likely to make cognitive errors or distortions characterized by a negative bias in the interpretation of facts when faced with perceived or real threating events, novel or ambiguous tasks (33). Whilst, at long term, negative effects act by decreasing scholastic performance and self-image (2). Anxiety complaints are frequently co-associated with depressive symptoms with rates ranging from 16 to 50% increasing in chronicity and severity (34, 35).

Based on these issues, critical uninvestigated question remains on the lack of a heterogenous assessment protocol to measure simultaneously different components of functioning in BIF pupils. Bridging this gap, this study aims to compare learning, motor and mental health profiles endorsed by pupils with borderline intellectual functioning and average intellectual functioning. The following hypotheses will be tested in this research:

- Hypothesis 1. Pupils with BIF would show worse learning profile compared with typically functioning peers by having lower performance on reading, writing and calculation tasks.
- Hypothesis 2. Pupils with BIF would perform poorly compared with AIF children on motor tasks.

- Hypothesis 3. Pupils with BIF would have lower scores on self-esteem at school and higher levels of school anxiety, depressed mood and insecurity than peers with AIF.

OUR STUDY

Participants were 38 children whose mean age was 9.28 yrs. (range 8-11 yrs; *SD* = .664). All children were attending fourth grade of the primary school and fell into two groups on the basis of level of intelligence: 1) Borderline intellectual functioning (BIF); 2) Average intellectual functioning (AIF). The BIF group was composed of 19 children (10 boys and 9 girls) with IQ scores ranging from 70 to 85. The AIF group, was composed by 19 children (9 boys and 10 girls) with IQ scores from 35 to 75th percentile. All children were in the fourth grade of primary school. There were no significant differences between the groups' average age ($p = .81$) or the average BMI ($p = .41$).

Prior to the start of the study, the approvals of the school heads and of the local ethical committee were obtained. Written informed consent was provided by each participant's parents. BIF and AIF children were recruited in their mainstream school on the basis of their intellectual functioning as previously assessed (2). They were administered a whole battery of tests aimed at measuring: 1. School profile; 2. Motor profile; 3. Mental Health profile.

School profile

The reading comprehension (36) measured pupils' reading comprehension of a story followed by 10 multiple-choice questions relating to the characters and events mentioned in the story. Participants were asked to choose the correct answer according to their understanding of the story. For each question, evaluation was binary, with a mark of 1 being attributed to each correct answer and 0 to incorrect items. Typical performance was 5 or more correct answers. Internal consistency reliability was a coefficient responding α = .60.

The reading decoding test (36) measured pupils' reading decoding. Given a text for each school level, children were required to read aloud a text within a 4-min time limit. Two parameters were evaluated: the number and the kind of errors by separate scores for accuracy and speed. As regard to accuracy, a score of 1 was assigned for each long pause or addition or omission of syllables, words, or lines. A score of 0.5 was attributed for each error of accent shift, hesitation, or self-correction. Normal performance was 6 or less errors. As regard to speed, the total score was obtained by seconds/syllables of read text. Average performance was score of 80 or less. Internal consistency reliability values were coefficient α of .75 and .64 for accuracy and speed respectively.

The word and nonword reading test (37) assessed accuracy and speed in reading tasks on words. It was composed of six 30 item lists: short word with high frequency of use, long word with high frequency of use, short word with low frequency of use, long word with low frequency of use, short nonword and long nonword. As regard to accuracy, the score 1 was given for each error. The speed was the time of execution indicated in seconds. The raw data thus obtained were eventually transformed into standard scores through tables in the manual.

The AC-MT test (38) measured multiple components of mathematical ability through collectively or individually administered tasks: number ordering (e.g., 36, 15, 276, 154), choice of the greatest number (e.g., 856, 428), written (e.g., 42 + 7) and oral computation (e.g., 28 X 4), number recall and processing (e.g., 7 x 8 in 4-5 seconds) and direct/indirect counting (e.g., counting aloud from 50 to 100 or from 100 to 50). Oral computation, number recall and processing and direct/indirect counting were individually administered. Four scores were obtained: 1. written calculation given by the sum of all correct items at calculation tasks; 2. number knowledge given by the sum of all correct performances at number ordering, choice of numbers… ; 3. accuracy given by the sum of errors at each individual task; 4. speed given by the sum of times at each individual task. The test-retest reliability of the battery ranged from .60 to .85.

Motor profile

Height and body weight were measured according to standardized practices recommended at the Airlie Conference (39). Body mass index (BMI) was calculated as body weight divided by height squared (kg/m^{-2}).

The TGM-Test of gross-motor development (20) measured pupils' gross motor development through two skill sets: locomotion and object control skills. Locomotion tasks required children to run as fast as possible for 15 meters, gallop for 10 meters, hop on one leg for 5 meters, jump forward, do a long jump, and take little jumps forward and laterally. Whilst object control tasks required children to catch a ball with a tennis racket, bounce off the ball, catch a ball, kick the ball running, and throw a ball with the hand. Based on the examiner's manual guidelines, participants were required to repeat each trial three times and a score of 1 was assigned if subject reached a good performance twice; a score of 0 was given when the child underperformed the item.

Two locomotion and object control raw total scores (maximum total score: 48) were computed by adding the items pertaining to each scale and then transformed into standard scores. Moreover a global gross motor quotient (GMQ) was obtained by adding the two partial scores. A GMQ ranging from 90 to 110 was average. The reliability was of $\alpha = .96$ for locomotion subtest and $\alpha = .97$ for object control subtest.

Mental health profile

The TMA-Multidimensional test of self-esteem (40) measured global self-worth by six subscales of self-esteem: Social, competence, affect, school, family and physical. In this study only the school subscale was used. It consisted of 25 items, positive and negative, investigating the way pupils feel about themselves in the school domain (e.g., "*I am proud of my school work*" or "*I do not understand much what I read*"). Pupils were asked to indicate to what extent each of the items corresponded to their self-perception on a 4 point Likert scale ranging from 1 (*Absolutely false*) to 4

(*Absolutely true*). A raw score was computed by summing the ratings given to each item and then transformed into standard score. A standard score ranging from 86 to 115 was average. The test-retest reliability of the battery was from $r = .90$.

SAFA-Self administrated psychiatric scales for children and adolescents (41) aimed at assessing mental impairments in children and adolescents with age ranging from 8 to 18 years. Specifically, SAFA was a battery that consisted of 6 clinical subscales: anxiety (SAFA A), depression (SAFA D), obsessive–compulsive symptoms (SAFA O), somatic symptoms and hypochondria (SAFA S), phobias (SAFA F) and Psychogenic eating disorders (SAFA P). Each subscale was suitable to be administrated separately from the others. Only SAFA A and SAFA D subscales were administered in this study. SAFA A measured the school anxiety and was composed of 12 items describing pupils' emotions related to school concerns (e.g., "*When I go to school I often feel very nervous*"). Children were asked to rate, using the 3-point scale from True to False how much they experienced each of described emotions. SAFA D measured the depressed mood by 6 items (e.g., *I often feel sad without any reason*) and the insecurity by 6 items (e.g., *I am self-confident).* Each item was presented on a 3-point scale from true to false. Total scores for SAFA A and SAFA D were computed by summing the ratings to each subscale. By using tables reported in the Examiner's Manual, raw scores were transformed into standard scores and percentile ranks. The cut-off of atypical emotional profile was of 70 standard score. The test-retest reliability of the battery was of $r = .90$.

Data analysis

Analyses of covariance (ANCOVA) were performed to compare learning, motor and emotional outcomes for BIF and AIF groups. The independent variable was intellectual level (BIF or AIF) and the covariate was the participants' gender. For all statistical tests the level of significance was set at $p < 0.05$. The SPSS Software (Version 20 for Windows) was adopted.

FINDINGS

With regard the learning profile, analyses revealed significant differences for reading comprehension [$F(1, 37) = 4.85$; $p = .034$, η^2 $p = .122$] and reading speed [$F(1, 37) = 4.280$; $p= .046$, η^2 $p = .109$], but not for reading accuracy [$F(1, 37) = 1.125$; $p = .29$, η^2 $p = .031$]. Pupils with BIF underscored on reading comprehension but showed higher speed compared to pupils with AIF.

Whilst, differences among the two groups were found on word and nonword reading tasks both as concern accuracy (Short nonword: [$F(1, 37) = 6.900$; $p = ,013$, η^2 $p = .165$]; Long nonword: [$F(1, 37) = 9.649$; $p = .004$, η^2 $p = .216$]; Long word with high frequency of use: [$F(1, 37) = 10.570$; $p = .003$, η^2 $p = .232$]; Short word with low frequency of use: [$F(1, 37) = 4.850$; $p = .034$, η^2 $p = .122$]; Long word with low frequency of use: [$F(1, 37) = 6.913$; $p = .013$, η^2 $p = .1652$]) and speed (Short word with high frequency of use: [$F(1, 37) = 5.324$; $p = .027$, η^2 $p = .132$]; Long word with high frequency of use: [$F(1, 37) = 9.313$; $p = .004$, η^2 $p = .219$]; Short word with low frequency of use: [$F(1, 37) = 8.031$; $p = .008$, η^2 $p = .187$]; Long word with low frequency of use: [$F(1, 37) = 6.913$; $p = .013$, η^2 $p = .165$]) with the BIF group having worse performance in all cases. Pupils in the BIF group showed more errors, on word and non word reading than those in the AIF group.

Pupils with BIF were always slower to read words and nonwords compared to AIF. Finally, as concern calculation outcomes, the BIF group differed significantly from the AIF group on written calculation [$F(1, 37) = 5.948$; $p = .020$, η^2 $p = .145$], number knowledge [$F(1, 37) = 9.505$; $p = .004$, η^2 $p = .214$], accuracy [$F(1, 37) = 6.387$; $p = .016$, η^2 $p = .154$] and speed [$F(1, 37) = 7.051$; $p = .012$, η^2 $p = .168$] with BIF pupils showing worse performance on written calculation and number knowledge as well as they showed more errors in accuracy and lower speed compared to AIF pupils (see Table 1).

Table 1. Descriptive statistics for learning profile measures as a function of group

Measures	BIF pupils (N = 19) M SD		AIF pupils (N = 19) M SD	
Reading comprehension	7.26	1.48	8.32	1.41
Reading accuracy	3.61	3.03	2.66	2.47
Reading speed	3.01	1.04	3.64	0.84
Short nonword accuracy	4.63	3.99	2	2.05
Short nonword speed	32.63	9.9	27.95	5.99
Long nonword accuracy	7.89	4.41	4.41	2.88
Long nonword speed	55.68	13.75	50	11.87
HFU short word accuracy	1.57	.58	.58	.59
HFU short word speed	25.63	8.61	20.47	4.66
HFU long word accuracy	2.58	.63	.84	.86
HFU long word speed	38.89	13.49	28.63	6.78
LFU short word accuracy	3.74	3.75	1.95	1.03
LFU short word speed	30.74	9.48	24.05	4.89
LFU long word accuracy	6.74	4.52	3.89	2.81
LFU long word speed	58.42	19.83	44.11	12.12
Written calculation	4.47	3.01	6.42	2.06
Number knowledge	14.74	6.22	19.42	3.17
Calculation accuracy	12.58	9.14	6.84	5.65
Calculation speed	202.89	116.21	141	59.57

Note: HFU short word speed = Short word with high frequency of use; HFU long word speed = Long word with high frequency of use; LFU short word = Short word with low frequency of use; LFU long word = Long word with low frequency of use.

With regard the motor profile, the two groups differed significantly on Gross Motor Quotient [$F(1, 37) = 15.013$; $p = .000$, η^2 $p = .300$] with the BIF group showing worse motor competence than AIF group.

As concern the subtests, group differences were found on both the Locomotion subtest [$F(1, 37)= 9,616$; $p = ,004$, η^2 $p = .216$] and the Object Control subtest [$F(1, 37) = 6.537$; $p = .015$, η^2 $p = .157$] BIF pupils performed poorly compared with AIF pupils (see Table 2).

Finally, with regard the mental health profile significant group differences were found for three of the 4 measures: school anxiety [$F(1, 37) = 5.039$; $p = .032$, η^2 $p = .140$], depressed mood [$F(1, 37) = 7.706$; $p = .009$, η^2 $p = .100$] and self-esteem [$F(1, 37) = 4.917$; $p = .034$,

η^2 p = .137]. To be more precise, the BIF group revealed higher levels of school anxiety and depressed mood and lower self-esteem than the AIF group (see Table 3).

Table 2. Descriptive statistics for motor profile measures as a function of group

Measures	BIF pupils (N = 19)		AIF pupils (N = 19)	
	M	SD	M	SD
BMI	19.28	3.44	18.36	3.68
GMQ	81.92	11.75	94.87	9.99
Locomotion skills	6.89	2.45	9	1.60
Object Control skills	7.47	2.93	9.63	2.65

Note: BMI = Body Mass Index; GMQ = Gross Motor Quotient.

Table 3. Descriptive statistics for mental health profile measures as a function of group

Measures	BIF pupils (N = 18)		AIF pupils (N = 19)	
	M	SD	M	SD
Self-Esteem	96	16.67	105.89	8.45
School anxiety	58.31	11.38	49.67	12.33
Depression mood	52.50	10.35	44.28	7.06
Insecurity	54.81	10.75	47.33	12.28

Discussion

The current study provided a comprehensive and multifaceted overview of functioning abilities in pupils with BIF compared to typically developing children. Three area processes have been investigated as being equally essential to function socially adaptively in every-day life: learning, movement and mental health.

First, as concern the learning profile, significant differences were found for reading comprehension and reading speed. In detail, BIF pupils demonstrated worse ability to comprehend events and characters of a written story than AIF peers. This is a well documented result and corroborated by ample literature demonstrating how abilities to process in deep events and understand written events is a function of higher intellectual level.

Surprisingly the results show BIF pupils to be quicker to read words in a text than AIF. However, this result is not contradictory with current literature demonstrating BIF condition to be characterized by general slowness (12, 14). When we analyze our groups' performances on word and nonword reading tasks, pupils with BIF spent more time to read short words with high frequency of use, long words with high frequency of use, short words with low frequency of use and long words with low frequency of use. In BIF condition longer time was required by short and long words irrespective of their frequency of use. Whilst, using nonword reading task similar performances among BIF and AIF pupils were obtained being unfamiliar, irregular stimuli and increasing in difficulty for both groups. This would be supposed as a ceiling effect which decreases performance of AIF pupils. Moreover, in interpreting the lack of differences among the two groups on reading accuracy performance as a function of the facilitating passage context, we argue that word and nonword reading task would be used as a pure measure of reading processing in a transparent orthography language as Italian (42). According to this view different performances among groups on these tasks can be interpreted. Pupils in the BIF group, compared to AIF, showed worse reading accuracy making significantly more errors on short and long nonwords, long words with high frequency of use, short and long words with low frequency of use. It is argued that unfamiliar and more difficult words, such as nonwords, words with low occurrence or long words, eliminate the frequency and semantic priming effects and allow to measure differences in reading as a function of the intellectual level.

Finally, as concern mathematical area, the BIF group exhibited significantly lower abilities on written calculation, number knowledge and accuracy as well as major slowness in calculation. Consistently, increasing research demonstrated the co-occurrence among BIF condition and specific deficits in calculation (7, 8, 15).

Taken together, these results corroborate findings previously obtained which highlighted impaired scholastic functioning as difficulties in reading, writing and calculation (1, 5, 8, 9). The link between intellectual functioning and school achievement is not direct, but it is mediated by domain-specific abilities playing a key role in sustaining and maintaining the readiness to learn. Weaken abilities on working memory, planning, attention and concentration can be conjectured to provide an explanation of the above-mentioned school difficulties (12-14).

Moreover, our results provided evidence for differences among groups on motor profile. BIF pupils got a gross motor quotient significantly below the mean value. They performed poorly on locomotion and object control tasks, compared with AIF pupils.

There were similarities between this motor profile and that outlined by previous work in this field underlining impaired gross-motor skills in children with borderline and mild intellectual disability (18, 19). The interplay between intellectual abilities and motor abilities in typical and atypical population has been well documented and explained by several reasons: the simultaneous stimulation of prefrontal cortex, cerebellum and basal ganglia by new and challenging motor tasks; a similar motor and cognitive developmental timetable showing a critical increase between 5 and 10 years; common underlying processes as inhibition, planning and monitoring (22, 23). However, our results are in contrast with previous findings revealing less impaired skills on the locomotor area than object-control skills in population with BIF to mild intellectual disability matched to TDC (18). In our BIF group no differences were found among locomotor skills such as walking, running, hopping, galloping, jumping, sliding or leaping and object-control skills such as throwing, catching, striking, bouncing, kicking, pulling or pushing.

Finally, as concern the mental health profile, BIF pupils demonstrated to have a lower level of self-esteem and, conversely, higher levels of school anxiety and depression mood. This result is consistent with previous studies demonstrating that anxiety complaints are the most common mental disorders affecting typical and atypical children and are in co-morbidity with depressive symptoms with rates from 16 to 50% (31, 34). Ample evidence has been produced highlighting low rates of school self-esteem and self-concept in condition of intellectual functioning below the median IQ (25, 32). Both adults and children who experienced repeated failure, such as those with BIF, are more likely to have higher levels of anxiety and depression compared to typically developing peers (28, 29, 31). This can result in withdrawal, self-defense and self-devaluation interfering with daily functioning and increasing in chronicity and severity (34, 35).

Implications

The main strength of this study lies in contributing to the current literature with respect to the planning of assessment in BIF condition. To date, assessment programs addressing domain-specific abilities has been developed. So, in current study a multidimensional and heterogeneous assessment protocol was implemented by integrating sessions aimed to measure learning, motor and mental health profiles. This arises by research evidence showing the equal load of school outcomes, motor skills and mental health in influencing and determining the intellectual and adaptive functioning of individuals with BIF. However, our data need to be carefully interpreted because they derived from the analysis of limited sample size weakening the generalizability of the current findings.

Notwithstanding this limitation, our study suggests some interesting implications for researchers and practitioners on the clinical and educational field for future practice. This can be used to implement targeted evidence-based intervention programs taking account both the specificity of disability and heterogeneous components influencing the functioning in BIF pupils.

To the best of our knowledge, no multifaceted program has been developed yet to improve simultaneously school and motor abilities or control anxiety and depressive risk factors which may cause or exacerbate underachievement and social-emotional maladjustments.

REFERENCES

[1] American Psychiatric Association. Diagnostic and statistical manual of mental disorders, 5th ed. Arlington, VA: American Psychiatric Association, 2013.

[2] Vianello R. Bisogni Educativi Speciali: il Funzionamento Intellettivo Limite o Borderline. Parma: Edizioni Junior, 2014. [Italian].

[3] Ninivaggi FJ. Borderline intellectual functioning in children and adolescents re-examining an underrecognized yet prevalent clinical comorbidity. Connecticut Med 2001;65:7–11.

[4] Peltopuro M, Ahonen T, Kaartinen J, Seppälä H, Närhi V. Borderline intellectual functioning: A systematic literature review. Intellect Dev Disabil 2014;52(6):419-43. doi:10.1352/1934-9556-52.6.419.

[5] Cornoldi C, Giofrè D, Orsini A, Pezzuti L. Differences in the intellectual profile of children with intellectual vs. learning disability. Res Dev Disabil 2014;35:2224–30. doi:10.1016/j.ridd.2014.05.013.

[6] Di Blasi FD, Savelli E, Zingale M, Buono S, Di Nuovo S. Effects of treatment of reading skills in a child with borderline intellectual functioning. Int J Disabil Hum Dev 2014;13(1):25-32. doi:10.1515/ijdhd-2013-0012.

[7] Jansen BRD, De Lange E, Van der Molen M. Math practice and its influence on math skills and executive functions in adolescents with mild to borderline intellectual disability. Res Dev Disabil 2013;34(5):1815-24. doi.10.1016/ j.ridd.2013.02.022.

[8] Salvador-Carulla L, García-Gutiérrez JC, Ruiz Gutiérrez-Colosía M, Artigas-Pallarès J, García Ibáñez J, et al. Borderline intellectual functioning: consensus and good practice guidelines. Rev Psiquiatr Salud Ment 2013;6:109–20. doi: 10.1016/j.rpsm.2012.12.001.

[9] Karande S, Kanchan S, Kulkarni M. Clinical and psychoeducational profile of children with borderline intellectual functioning. Indian J Pediatr 2008;75(8):795-800. doi:10.1007/s12098-008-0101-y.

[10] Istituto Superiore di Sanità (ISS), Sistema Nazionale Linee Guida, Consensus Conference Disturbi Specifici di Apprendimento, 2011. URL: http://snlg–iss.it/cc_disturbi_specifici_apprendimento.

[11] Alloway TP. Working memory and executive function profiles of individuals with borderline intellectual functioning. J Intellect Disabil Res 2010;54(5):448-56. doi:10.1111/j.1365-2788.2010.01281.x.

[12] Bonifacci P, Snowling MJ. Speed of processing and reading disability: A cross-linguistic investigation of dyslexia and borderline intellectual functioning. Cognition 2008;107:999–17. doi: 10.1016/j.cognition.2007.12.006.

[13] Schuchardt K, Gebhardt M, Maehler C. Working memory functions in children with different degrees of intellectual disability. J Intellect Disabil Res 2010;54:346-53. doi:10.1111/j.1365-2788.2010.01265.x.

[14] Van Nieuwenhuijzen M, Vriens A, Scheepmakerc M, Smitc M, Porton E. The development of a diagnostic instrument to measure social information processing in children with mild to borderline intellectual disabilities. Res Dev Disabil 2011;32:358–70. doi:10.1016/j.ridd.2010.10.012.

[15] Baglio F, Cabini M, Ricci C, Baglio G, Lipari S, Griffanti L, et al. Abnormal development of sensory-motor, visual temporal and parahippocampal cortex in children with learning disabilities and borderline intellectual functioning. Front Hum Neurosci 2014;8:806. doi:10.3389/fnhum.2014.00806.

[16] Simons J, Daly D, Theodorou F, Caron C, Simons J, Andoniadou E. Validity and reliability of the TGMD-2 in 7-10 year old Flemish children with intellectual disability. Adapt Phys Activ Q 2008;25:71-82. doi:10.1123/apaq.25.1.71.

[17] Vuijk PJ, Hartman E, Scherder E, Visscher C. Motor performance of children with mild intellectual disability and borderline intellectual functioning. J Intellect Disabil Res 2010;54:955–65. doi:10.1111/j.1365-2788.2010.01318.x.

[18] Hartman E, Houwen S, Scherder E, Visscher C. On the relationship between motor performance and executive functioning in children with intellectual disabilities. J Intellect Disabil Res 2010;54:468–77. doi:10.1111/j.1365-2788.2010.01284.x.

[19] Westendorp M, Houwen S, Hartman E, Visscher C. Are gross motor skills and sports participation related in children with intellectual disabilities? Res Dev Disabil 2011;32:1147–53. doi:10.1016/j.ridd.2011.01.009.

[20] Ulrich DA. Test of gross motor development. Austin, TX: Pro-ed Publishers, 1985 .

[21] Ulrich DA. Test of gross motor development, 2th edition Austin, TX: Pro-ed Publishers, 2000.

[22] Alesi M, Bianco A, Luppina G, Palma A, Pepi A Improving children's coordinative skills and executive functions: the effects of a football exercise program. Percept Mot Skills 2016;122(1):27–46 doi: 10.1177/0031512515627527.

[23] Shin I, Park EY. Meta-analysis of the effect of exercise programs for individuals with intellectual disabilities. Res Dev Disabil 2012;33:1937-47. doi: 10.1016/j.ridd.2012.05.019.

[24] Chen MD, Tsai HY, Wang CC, Wuang YP. The effectiveness of racket-sport intervention on visual perception and executive functions in children with mild intellectual disabilities and borderline intellectual functioning. Neuropsychiatr Dis Treat 2015;11:2287-97. doi:10.2147/NDT.S8908.

[25] Cooper S, Smiley E, Morrison J, Williamson A, Allan A. Mental ill-health in adults with intellectual disabilities: prevalence and associated factors. Br J Psychiatry 2007;190:27–35. doi:10.1192/bjp.bp.106.022483.

[26] Einfeld S, Piccinin AM, Mackinnon A, Hofer SM, Taffe J, Gray KM et al. Psychopathology in young people with intellectual disability. JAMA 2006;296(16):1981–89. doi:10.1001/jama.296.16.1981.

[27] Emerson E, Einfeld S, Stancliffe RJ. The mental health of young children with intellectual disabilities or borderline intellectual functioning. Soc Psychiatry Psychiatr Epidemiol 2010;45:579–87. doi:10.1007/s00127-009-0100-y.

[28] Emerson E, Hatton C The mental health of children and adolescents with intellectual disabilities in Britain. Br J Psychiatry 2007;191:493–9. doi:10.1192/bjp.bp.107.038729.

[29] Fernell E, Ek U. Borderline intellectual functioning in children and adolescents – insufficiently recognized difficulties. Acta Paediatr 2010;99:748–53. doi:10.1111/j.1651-2227.2010.01707.x.

[30] Grills-Taquechel AE, Fletcher JM, Vaughn SR, Stuebing KK. Anxiety and reading difficulties in early elementary school: evidence for unidirectional or bi-directional relations?. Child Psychiatry Hum Dev 2012;43(1):35-57. doi: 10.1007/s10578-011-0246-1.

[31] Alesi M, Rappo G, Pepi A. Emotional profile and intellectual functioning: A comparison among children with borderline intellectual functioning, average intellectual functioning and gifted intellectual functioning. SAGE Open 2015 Jul 13:1–9. doi:10.1177/2158244015589995.

[32] Majida RA, Alias A. Consequences of risk factors in the development of gifted children. Procedia Soc Behav Sci 2010;7:63–9. doi:10.1016/j.sbspro.2010.10.010.

[33] Pereira AIF, Barros L, Mendonça D. Cognitive errors and anxiety in school aged children. Psicologia 2012;25(4):817-23.

[34] Jacobson NC, Newman MG. Avoidance mediates the relationship between anxiety and depression over a decade later. J Anxiety Disord 2014;28(5):437-45. doi: 10.1016/j.janxdis.2014.03.007.

[35] Wright M, Banerjee R, Hoek W, Rieffe C, Novin S. Depression and social anxiety in children: Differential links with coping strategies. J Abnorm Child Psychol 2010;38:405–19. doi:10.1007/s10802-009-9375-4.

[36] Cornoldi C, Colpo G. Prove oggettive MT di lettura. Firenze: Organizzazioni Speciali, 2001. [Italian]

[37] Zoccolotti P, De Luca M, Di Filippo G, Judica A, Spinelli D. Prova di lettura di parole e non parole. Roma: Fondazione Santa Lucia IRCCS, 2005. [Italian]

[38] Cornoldi C, Lucangeli D, Bellina M. Test AC-MT 6-11.Test di Valutazione delle Abilità di Calcolo. Trento: Edizioni Erickson, 2005. [Italian]

[39] Lohman TG, Roche AF, Martorell R. Anthropometric standardization reference manual. Champaign, IL: Human Kinetics, 1988.

[40] Bracken BA. MSCS Multidimensional Self-Concept Scale. Austin, TX: Pro-ed, 1992.

[41] Cianchetti C, Fancello GS. SAFA Scale Psichiatriche di Autosomministrazione per Fanciulli e Adolescenti. Firenze: Organizzazioni Speciali, 2001. [Italian]

[42] Paizi D, Burani C, Zoccolotti O. List context effects in reading Italian words and nonwords: can the word frequency effect be eliminated? Eur J Cogn Psychol. 2010;22(7):1039-65. doi:10.1080/09541440903216492.

In: Intellectual Disability
Editors: Ariel Tenenbaum et al.
ISBN: 978-1-53617-866-1

Chapter 8

EFFECTS OF SOCIAL SKILLS TRAINING USING TEACHING STRATEGIES FROM APPLIED BEHAVIOUR ANALYSIS ON THE SOCIAL DEVELOPMENT OF CHILDREN WITH MILD AND MODERATE INTELLECTUAL DISABILITIES

Ritu Kalgotra**, PhD and Jaspal S Warwal, PhD
Department of Education, University of Jammu, Jammu, India

ABSTRACT

The present research aimed to study the effect of social skills training using the strategies from Applied Behavior Analysis on the social skills of children with mild and moderate intellectual disabilities at special schools of an Indian state. In a non-randomized pre-test post-test control group design, children with mild (n = 34) and moderate (n = 36)

*Corresponding Author's E-mail: ritusatya7@rediffmail.com.

intellectual disabilities were placed into control and experimental group. Both the groups were tested with Social Skills Rating Scale devised by the researchers as a pre-test and as a post-test after intervention in social skills training to the experimental group. ANCOVA analysis indicated $F(1, 31) = 287.13$, $P = .00$ for the children with mild intellectual disabilities, $F(1, 33) = 127.55$, $P = .00$ for the children with moderate intellectual disabilities on Social Skill Rating Scale. Social skills training using teaching strategies from Applied Behaviour Analysis is an effective intervention for improving their social skills in all the domains of Social Skills Rating Scale. The program can be introduced at special schools in the daily curriculum to improve the social skills of the children with mild and moderate intellectual disabilities.

INTRODUCTION

Deficits in social skills are key criteria in defining high-incidence of intellectual disabilities (1). Skills such as communication, problem-solving and decision-making, assertion, group interaction, and self-management (2) help to initiate and maintain positive social relationships with peers, teachers, family and other community members (3). These skills also help in building satisfying relationships, receiving positive feedbacks (4), preventing the negative ones and facilitating interpersonal relationships (5). Deficits in social skills frequently co-occur with intellectual disability (6), which is often manifested as delays in effective communication and social interaction, with impairments demonstrated across communication partners (7-8). Lack of social skills limits opportunities for meaningful social interaction, acceptance by peers, and classroom performance (9). Due to the deficiency in social skills, individuals with intellectual disabilities face difficulty interacting with their peers (10-11) and adjusting behaviours which is a constraint for them to have mutual relationships with others. These children have inadequacies in social skills, such as helping one another, sharing and exchanging greetings (11) and therefore, can exhibit problematic behaviors (5). Educational programs at Indian special schools focus on functional academics, daily living skills, and vocational training and little emphasis is on the development of their social skills. But, the aim of training for individuals with intellectual disabilities is to prepare them for social life (12). Therefore, present research aimed to study the effects of social skills training program developed by the researchers on the social skills of the children with mild and moderate intellectual disabilities at the special schools.

Hypotheses

- There is no significant difference in the adjusted mean scores of social skills of experimental and control groups children with mild intellectual disabilities by considering Pre-social skills as a covariate.
- There is no significant difference in the adjusted mean scores of social skills of experimental and control groups children with moderate intellectual disabilities by considering Pre-social skills as a covariate.

OUR STUDY

In quasi-experimental research, pre-test post-test control group design was used where participants were placed into experimental and control groups non-randomly. Participants were not randomly matched to the experimental and control groups because the sample was small. Moreover, disturbing children from their natural environment could also have caused inconvenience thereby reducing the effectiveness of the intervention. Studying children in their natural setting had an advantage of increased degree of external validity of the research. The children with mild and moderate intellectual disabilities at three selected special schools were placed into experimental groups and the children of two schools were placed into the control groups. So, four non-equivalent groups of children with mild and moderate intellectual disabilities were formed where children with mild intellectual disabilities were placed in the experimental and control groups forming two groups and similarly children with moderate intellectual disabilities were also placed into experimental and control groups. Differences in these non-equivalent groups due to non-randomization were controlled during the statistical analysis.

Ethical considerations

Ethical approval was obtained from Department of Education, University of Jammu. The permission from the head of the institution was granted to conduct research. Participants were assured that their identities and personal information would remain confidential during reporting of the study. The study procedure was explained in detail through information forms to the legal guardians who then signed the consent forms.

Selection criteria

The inclusion criteria followed while selecting the sample were presence of intellectual disability as per the International Classification of Diseases-10 (13) criteria, mild and moderate intellectual disabled children as identified by an IQ test, children in age range from 6 to 17 years, children following intervention procedures safely and children attending special schools five days per week for five hours a day. The exclusion criteria included current symptoms of cerebral palsy, physical disabilities, multiple disabilities, severe behaviour disorders or destructive behaviour and current use of sedative medication. Due to the poor response of the children with severe and profound intellectual disabilities to follow social skills training, they were also excluded.

Participant's recruitment and description of participants

At five special schools of Jammu district (Jammu and Kashmir, India), Seguin Form Board Intelligence test (14) was administered individually to all the children to determine their IQ. On the basis of their IQ scores, children were categorized into mild, moderate and severe intellectual disabilities as per the International Classification of Diseases-10 (13) criteria. Only children with mild and moderate intellectual disabilities fulfilling the selection criteria were selected for the study and placed into control and experimental groups as per research design.

The total sample comprised of seventy children with mild and moderate intellectual disabilities placed separately into control and experimental groups forming four non-equivalent groups. One female in the mild control group, one male and one female child from the moderate control group were autistic whereas two male children from the mild experimental group, three male and two females from the moderate control group and two male children from the moderate experimental group were children with Down syndrome. At the baseline, 73 children were selected but three children left the school due to the transfer of parents in their job. Total of 55.7% of the sample belonged to the urban area and 44.3% of the sample belonged to the rural area.

Intervention in social skills training

This intervention module was developed by the researchers after getting feedback from the caretakers, heads of institutions, teacher's approval to implement it. The module included teaching strategies, social skills, teaching procedure of each skill, and time schedule. Skills were taught under the supervision of two trained teachers who were trained for the different social skills, teaching strategies, time schedule, etc. by the researchers. To ensure replication of intervention program, the researchers used the TIDieR checklist and guide (15).

Time schedule

Social skill training intervention comprised of eight social skills where each skill was taught for three weeks for 60 minutes daily. After twenty-four weeks, all the skills were practiced for another eight weeks (total 32 weeks).

Teaching strategies

Social skills were taught to the experimental groups using teaching strategies adapted from Applied Behaviour Analysis such as verbal instruction, modeling, role-playing, prompting, rewards, and feedback. Single skill was taught at a time individually and in small groups to enhance sequencing and retention. Appropriate physical and verbal prompting was used to guide correct responses. Teachers always gave a positive response, praising each child's efforts and appropriately rewarded the desired behavior.

Social skills

1. Interactional skills: The interactional skills such as smiles in response to others, waving goodbye, greeting others, using magic words (thank you, sorry, please, excuse me), and returning borrowed materials were taught through modelling and then by role-playing.
2. Introducing skill: Children were instructed to introduce themselves at a food store/party through modelling and then by role-playing.
3. Friendship-making skill: The children were instructed how to start talking to others in a group and then the skill of making small talks was demonstrated through modelling and then by role-playing.
4. Phoning the relatives (father, mother, sister or brother): The skill how to start talking to their relatives on phone and expressing how

theyfeel in the school, what they have done last week and how they are doing in life was taught verbally, though modelling and then by role-playing to the children

5. Cleanliness skill: Teachers demonstrated cleanliness skills through modeling and then by role-playing. Cleanliness skills included washing hands, eating food calmly, not to talk while eating food, brush teeth after eating food, putting on clean clothes and folding clothes, combing hair daily, collecting wastes and throwing in the dustbin, and sweeping floor using a broom.
6. Health safety and security skill: Children were taught about the need for health safety and security skill through teaching strategies. Children were taught how to avoid playing with the matchstick, avoid playing on the top of walls and hills, and to avoid throwing the stones/things on others.
7. Aggression control skill: Children were taught how to be calm in every situation. The consequences of aggression were demonstrated through role-playing. The social skills taught included refraining from aggressive behaviour towards peers and self, allowing others to comfort him/her if upset or agitated, self-regulating when tense /upset or high energy, dealing with being left out of a group, accepting not being first at a game or activity, accepting losing at a game without becoming upset/angry, saying "no" in acceptable way to things he/she does not want to do, using appropriate voice tone and volume during talks.
8. Cooperative playing: Children were motivated to play in the group rather than alone. The skills included sharing toys and talks about the activity with peers even though the play agenda of the other children is different, physically and verbally responding to interactions from peers (accepts toy from peer, answers questions), knowing appropriate ways of joining in an activity with peers, inviting others to play, turn-taking during play activities, obeying game rules, requesting toys, food, and materials from peers, and playing cooperatively with peers during play.

Intervention fidelity

The intervention was well supervised and implemented as per the program, through a checklist which was prepared with the program which ensured timely completion of all the activities. A daily record all the activities was also maintained in the logbook by the teachers/supervisors. During the study, the researchers visited the special schools regularly to monitor the implementation of the intervention and provided feedback to further standardize the intervention. Moreover, there was no modification in the intervention program during the course of study. To ensure standardized delivery of training across all schools, all the teachers adhered to a single training protocol.

Data collection instruments

Seguin Form Board Test (14) was used to assess Intelligence Quotient through visual discrimination, matching, speed, accuracy, eye-hand coordination and visual-motor skills. It consists of ten geometrically shaped wooden blocks and a large form board with recessed corresponding shapes. The children were asked to match wooden blocks on the form board and place on their corresponding shapes. Test-retest was done after 20 days' time interval to check the reliability of the scale r (25) = 0.81.

Socio-economic status scale (16) was used to assess the socio-economic status of children in a society under of four areas as Finance, Property, Education and Social status. It is a point-scale; points ranging between 3 and 10 depending upon the component of the variable under assessment. Test-retest was done to find its reliability which was r (35) = .81, $P < .01$ with 30 days' time interval.

Social Skills Rating Scale

A 66- item Social Skills Rating was devised by the researchers and standardized on the sample to fifty-five children with mild and moderate intellectual disabilities at special schools of Jammu district of Jammu

&Kashmir (India). The mean baseline scores of social skills were *M*= 22.60, *SD*= 7.39 for Interactional skill, *M*= 6.34, *SD*= 1.62 for introducing skill, *M*= 12.52, *SD*= 5.22 for Friendship making skill, *M*= 5.56, *SD*= 3.05 for Phoning the relatives, *M*= 8.21, *SD*= 2.87 for Cleanliness skill, *M*= 2.36, *SD*= 1.43 for Health safety and security, *M*= 8.49, *SD*= 3.82 for Aggression control, *M*= 6.85, *SD*= 2.98 for Cooperative playing skill. The overall mean for all the domains were *M* = 72.96, SD = 19.56. The measures of reliability were calculated by Cronbach's Alpha, ($N = 55$) was 0.811 indicating very good reliability. Test-retest reliability ($N = 55$) was evaluated at intake and again after a mean duration of 4 months, which was $r\ (53) = .781$, $p < .05$ indicating good test-retest reliability. Due to the poor response of the children with severe and profound intellectual disabilities on Social Skills Rating Scale, it was standardized on the children with mild and moderate intellectual disabilities only.

Procedures

Parents/guardians were requested to provide information on the socio-economic status scale during the parent-teacher meeting. Social Skills Rating Scale was administered to both the control and experimental groups as the pre-test. Intervention in social skills training was introduced to the experimental group as explained in the training program in the selected schools of Jammu city for thirty-two weeks. Control group participants were not involved in any additional social skills activities. Assessment of social skills was done after thirty-two weeks (post-test) on the completion of intervention program through Social Skills Rating Scale on both the control and experimental groups. Social skills of each child were individually observed during the pre-testing and post-testing by the researchers.

Statistical analysis

Descriptive and inferential statistics were used to analyze and describe the data pertaining to Social Skills Rating Scale on children with mild and moderate intellectual disabilities. Means, standard deviation, and Analysis of Covariance were used to analyze the data. In the present research, pre-test scores are used as covariates in pre-test post-test control group quasi-experimental designs. It became difficult for us to match an equal number of children with mild and moderate intellectual disabilities on different criteria and to put them in experimental and control conditions at the same time randomly. ANCOVA was used to analyze data because it adjusts the post-test means due to non-randomization. With non-randomized designs, the main purpose of ANCOVA is to adjust the post-test means for differences among groups on the pre-test, because such differences are likely to occur with intact groups which keep the participants in natural settings, allowing a higher degree of external validity (17). ANCOVA is used in quasi-experiments when subjects cannot be assigned randomly to control and experimental groups (18).

FINDINGS

Table 1 shows the children with mild and moderate intellectual disabilities (Age, Intelligence Quotient and Socio-economic status) selected for intervention in social skills training. The overall scores on the Socio economic status scale were $N= 70$, $M= 60.742$, $SD= 11.084$. 1.4% of the total sample belonged to above average socio-economic status, 48.6% of the children belonged to average socio-economic status, 44.3% of the children belonged to below average socio-economic status and 5.7% of the children belonged to the poor socio-economic status.

Table 1. Characteristics of children with mild and moderate intellectual disabilities (Age, Intelligence Quotient) and socio-economic status selected for intervention in social skills training

Type of Group disability	Age (yrs)		I.Q		Socio-economic status (percentage)
	M	SD	M	SD	
Mild Control (n = 20)	13.66	3.14	58.85	4.82	30 (A), 70 (BA)
Experiment (n = 14)	12.13	2.99	57.40	3.42	70 (A), 30(BA)
Mod Control (n = 15)	12.61	2.92	42.57	3.22	33 (A), 70(BA), 20 (P)
Experiment (n = 21)	11.47	2.22	41.16	3.21	5(AA), 62 (BA), 5(P)

AA = Above Average, A = Average, BA = Below Average, P = Poor.

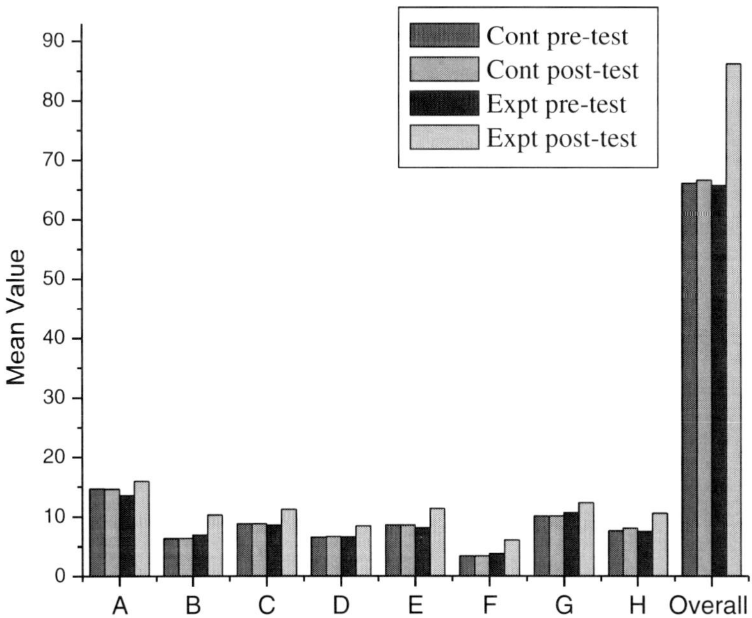

Figure 1. Comparison between pre-test and post-test scores of control and the experimental group of children with mild intellectual disabilities on different domains of Social Skills Rating Scale.

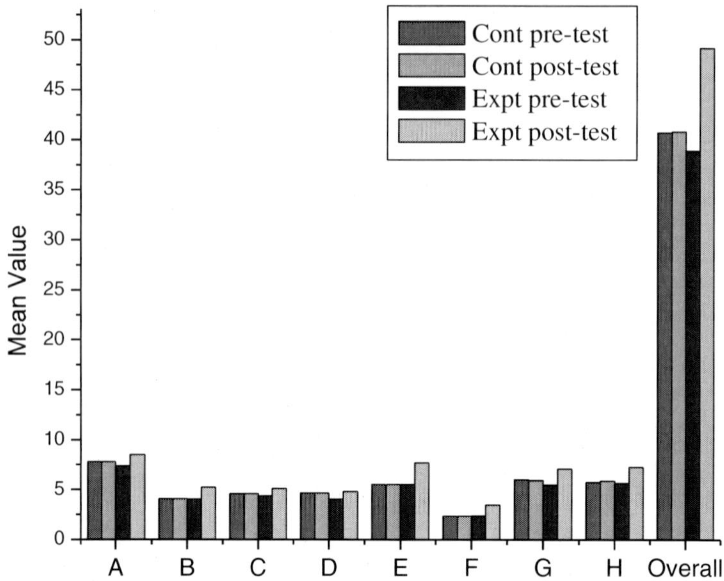

Figure 2. Comparison between pre-test and post-test scores of control and experiment group of children with moderate intellectual disabilities on different domains of Social Skills Rating Scale.

Table 2. Results of analysis of covariance in control group and the experimental group children with mild and moderate intellectual disabilities on Social Skills Rating Scale

Type of disability		**Sum of squares**	**df**	**Mean square**	**F**	***p***	**effect size**
Mild	Contrast	3264.86	1	3264.86	287.13*	.000	.903
	Error	352.48	31	11.37			
Mod	Contrast	895.39	1	895.39	127.55*	.000	.794
	Error	231.65	33	231.65			

* $P < .05$

The mean pre-test and post-test scores of different social skills of control and experimental groups children with mild and moderate intellectual disabilities on Social Skills Rating Scale are graphically represented in Figures 1 and 2. Comparing the mean scores of both the children with mild and moderate intellectual disabilities, it was found that the children with mild intellectual disabilities had higher post-test scores (mean) in experiment group as compared to children with moderate intellectual disabilities in all the domains of social skills. The mean pre-test scores of children with mild intellectual disabilities were higher than the children with moderate intellectual disabilities on both control and experiment groups which indicated that the children with mild intellectual disabilities had better social skills than children with moderate intellectual disabilities.

Results of Analysis of Covariance of children with mild intellectual disabilities on Social Skills Rating Scale (see Table 2) indicated that adjusted F (1, 31) = 287.13, P = .000 is significant at .01 level. The adjusted mean score of social skills of the experimental group was 86.33, which is significantly higher than that of the control group whose adjusted mean score was 66.41(see Figure 3). Thus, the null hypothesis "There is no significant difference in the adjusted mean scores of social skills of control and experimental groups children with mild intellectual disabilities by considering Pre-social skills as a covariate" is rejected. Since a significant difference was found in the adjusted mean scores of social skills of control and experimental group, the effect size was also calculated. The effect size for the intervention in social skills training on the children with mild intellectual disabilities was .903 which indicated large effect of the intervention (see Table 2).

Similarly, in children with moderate intellectual disabilities, adjusted F (1, 33) = 127.55, P = .000 is significant at .01 level. The adjusted mean score of social skills of the experimental group was 49.926, which is significantly higher than that of the control group whose adjusted mean score was 39.703 (see Figure 3). Thus, the null hypothesis "There is no significant difference in the adjusted mean scores of social skills of control and experimental groups children with moderate intellectual disabilities by considering Pre-social skills as a covariate" is rejected. The effect size for the intervention in social skills training on the children with moderate intellectual disabilities was 0.794 which indicated a medium effect of the intervention (see Table 2).

Table 3.Results of Analysis of Covariance of different domains of social skills of the children with mild and moderate intellectual disabilities on Social Skills Rating Scale

Type of disability	Social skills	df	F	p	Effect size
Mild A	Interactional skills	1,31	102.67*	. 000	.768
B	Introducing skills	1,31	94.66*	.000	.753
C	Friendship making skill	1,31	62.24*	.000	.663
D	Phoning the relatives	1,31	87.520*	.000	.738
E	Cleanliness skill	1,31	73.35*	.000	.703
F	Health safety and Security	1,31	65.65*	.000	.679
G	Aggression control	1,31	61.89*	.000	.666
H	Cooperative playing	1, 33	117.29*	.000	.791
Mod A	Interactional skills	1,33	46.039*	.000	.582
B	Introducing skills	1,33	56.53*	.000	.631
C	Friendship making skill	1,33	12.82*	.001	.280
D	Phoning the relatives	1,33	16.26*	.000	.330
E	Cleanliness skill	1,33	47.93*	.186	.592
F	Health safety and Security	1,33	17.55*	.001	.347
G	Aggression control	1,33	27.56*	.000	.455
H	Cooperative playing	1,33	67.38	.000	.671

* $P < .05$

Results indicated that intervention in social skills training produced significant changes in the domains of Interactional skills F (1,31) = 102.67, P = .000, Introducing skill F (1,31) = 94.66, P = .000, Friendship making skill F (1,31) = 62.24, P = .000, Phoning the relatives F (1,31) = 87.52, P = .000, Cleanliness Skill F (1,31) = 73.35, P = .000, Health safety and security F (1,31) = 65.65, P = .000, Aggression Control F (1,31) = 61.89, P = .000, Cooperative playing F (1,31) = 117.29, P = .000, of children with mild intellectual disability but their control group did not show any significant difference in these domains of social skills (see Table 3). Similarly, intervention in social skills training produced significant changes in the domains of Interactional skills F (1,33) = 46.03, P = .000, Introducing skill F (1,33) = 56.53, P = .000, Friendship making skill F (1,33) = 12.82, P = .000, Phoning the relatives F (1,33) = 16.26, P = .000,

Cleanliness Skill F (1,33) = 47.93, P = .000, Health safety and security F (1,33) = 17.55, P = .000, Aggression Control F (1,33) = 27.56, P = .000 and Cooperative playing F (1,33) = 67.38, P = .000 of children with moderate intellectual disability but their control group did not show any significant difference in these domains of social skills.

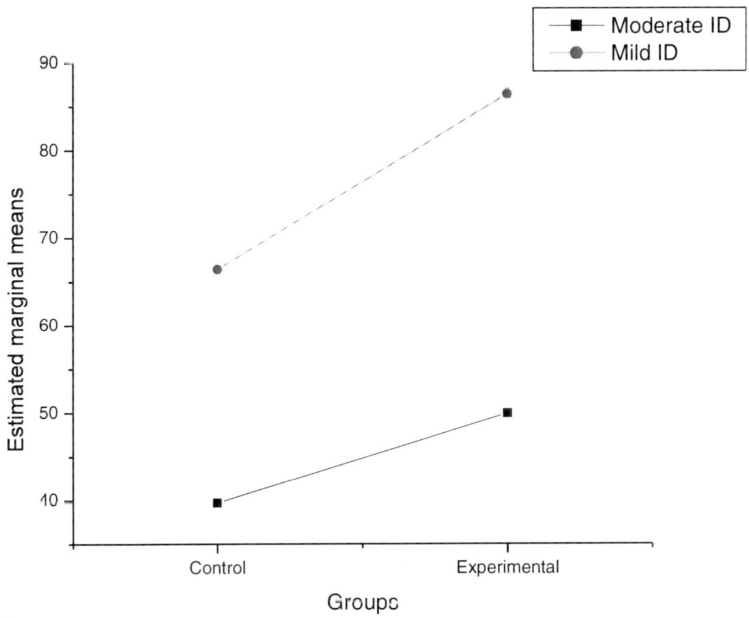

Figure 3. Graphical representation of estimated marginal mean of post-test of children with mild and moderate intellectual disabilities on Social Skills Rating Scale.

Comparing the effect size of the intervention in social skills training through Social Skills Rating Scale of the children with mild and moderate intellectual disabilities, it was found that the children with mild intellectual disabilities had higher effect size as compared to children with moderate intellectual disabilities in all the domains of social skills (see Table 3). The results reflected that there is a significant effect of social skills training on the social skills of the children with mild and moderate intellectual disabilities when both control and experimental groups were matched with pre-social skills scores.

DISCUSSION

It was inferred that Social skills training using teaching strategies from Applied Behaviour Analysis is an effective intervention for improving social skills in all the domains of social skills among children with mild and moderate intellectual disabilities at special schools in India.

The similarity of present research in methodology with that of other researchers is discussed here. Tekinarslan and Sucuoglu (19) indicated that cognitive-process approach based social skills program was effective on learning and generalizing three social skills (apologizing, coping with teasing and avoiding inappropriate touching) of the nine students with intellectual disabilities. Bates (20) studied the effectiveness of interpersonal skills training on the communication skill acquisition of sixteen children with moderate and mild intellectual disabilities through instructions in the introduction and small talk, providing play materials and interacting with children during play. The instructional package included verbal instruction, modeling, role-playing, and feedback which are similar to the present study. Alavi, Savoji and Amin (21) investigated the effect of social skills training on the aggression of children with intellectual disabilities where the experimental group was trained in social skills for two hours, and the performance of the two groups was compared in the pre-test and post-test. Pasha and Gorjian (22) examined the effect of training social skills on social development through administering Vineland's social development instrument on seventy persons with intellectual disabilities as a pretest and posttest.

Teaching strategies as adopted from Applied Behavior Analysis in the present research were also used by Matson et al. (23) where three autistic children and children with intellectual disabilities were taught shoe tying, tooth brushing, hair combing, putting on pants, shirt, and socks, and eating and drinking by using modeling, verbal instructions, prompting, edible and social reinforcement. Leblanc, and Matson (24) assessed a social skills training program with 32 developmentally delayed preschoolers where the treatment group was trained for 6-week protocol involving positive reinforcement, modeling, rehearsal, feedback, and timeout. Yakubova and

Taber-Doughty (25) taught three students with autism to engage in a series of social skills through the use of video modeling and verbal prompting once during each intervention session for three weeks. Bielecki and Swender (26) indicated that behavioral observations and role-playing are common methods for assessing social skills.

In the present research, social skills program included social skills in different domains such as interactional skills, introducing skills, friendship making skill, phoning the relative, cleanliness skill, health safety and security, aggression control, cooperative playing skill which are similar to social skills used by Tekinarslan, and Sucuoglu (19) such as social coding skills, social decision skills, social performance skills and social evaluation skills to teach targeted social skills.

The present research concluded that there is significant effect of social skills training on children with mild and moderate intellectual disabilities at special schools which is supported by different authors. A similar conclusion was given by Salomon (27) that one of the most effective treatment methods for these children were training social skills. Pasha, and Gorjian (22) indicated significant differences between the experimental and control group on social development. O'Handley et al. (28) concluded that all participants demonstrated improvements in skill accuracy, with teacher ratings of social functioning in a study evaluating the effects of the Superheroes Social Skills program. Tekinarslan and Sucuoglu (19) targeted social skills program was also effective for children with intellectual disabilities to acquire targeted social skills.

Implications of the study

Intervention in social skills training is an interesting, safe program that required trained teachers who could systematically implement it using teaching strategies from Applied Behaviour Analysis. This social skills training module can be introduced as a part of the daily curriculum at Indian special schools which can add fun-filled play and recreation activities in their daily routine. It is can also be tested on children and adults with behaviour disorders, destructive behaviour and as treatment of depression and anxiety. This training program engages them in more useful activities during the day and reduces their non-work activities through stimulating their cognitive, social and emotional development. Results of this study could be generalized to other Indian states with the similar cultural, geographical, social and political environment. The sample represented both rural and urban areas, and also different socio-economic status, which increases the ecological validity of the results.

Limitations of the study

The intervention was conducted at special schools in a restricted area within school hours. It was difficult to motivate some children as they lacked interest to take part in the social skills training. Reason for poor improvement in the social skills after training also required further research. The future researchers should conduct follow-up after the post-test to evaluate the retention of the learnt skill.

REFERENCES

[1] Gresham FM, Sugai G, Horner RH. Interpreting outcomes of social skills training for students with high-incidence disabilities. Except Child 2001;67(3):331-44.

[2] Haager D, Vaughn S. Parent, teacher, peer and self-reports of the social competence of students with learning disabilities. Except Child 1995;26:205-17.

[3] Quinn M M, Jannasch-Penell A, Rutherford RB. Using peers as social skills training agents for students with antisocial behavior. A cooperative learning approach. PrevSoc Failure 1995;39:26-31.

[4] Geldard K, Geldard D. Counselling children: A practical introduction, 3rd edition, London: Sage, 2008.

[5] Warger CL, Rutherford R. Social skills instruction: A collaborative approach. Washington, DC: Foundation Exceptional Innovations, 1996.

[6] Kavale KA, Forness SR. Social skill deficits and learning disabilities: A meta-analysis. J Learn Disabil 1996;29:226-37.

[7] Alwell M, Cobb B. Social and communicative interventions and transition outcomes for youth with disabilities: A systematic review. Career Dev Trans Except Individ 2009;32:94-107.

[8] Carter EW, Sisco LG, Chung Y, Stanton-Chapman TL. Peer interactions of students with intellectual disabilities and/or autism: A map of the intervention literature. Res Pract Persons Severe Disabil 2010;35:63-79.

[9] Siperstein GN, Parker RC, Norins Bardon J, Widaman KF. A national study of youth attitudes toward the inclusion of students with intellectual disabilities. Except Child 2007;73:435-55.

[10] Heiman T, Margalit M. Loneliness, depression, and social skills among students with mild mental retardation in different educational settings. J Spec Educ 1998; 32(3):154-63.

[11] Sargent LR. Social skills for school and community. Systematic instruction for children and youth with cognitive delay. Washington, DC: Division Mental Retardation Council Exceptional Children, 1991.

[12] Dever RB, Knapczyk DR. Teaching persons with mental retardation. A model for curriculum development and teaching. Boston, MA: McGraw Hill, 1997.

[13] World Health Organisation. Manual of the international classification of disease, injuries, and causes of death-10. Geneva: WHO, 1992.

[14] Venkatesan S. Revalidation of Seguin Form Board Test for Indian children. Indian J ApplPsychol 1998;35:38-42.

[15] Hoffmann TC, Glasziou PP, Boutron I, Milne R, Perera R, Moher D, et al. Better reporting of interventions: template for intervention description and replication (TIDieR) checklist and guide. BMJ 2014;348:1687. doi: 10.1136/bmj.g1687.

[16] Meenakshi. Manual for Socio Economic Status Scale. Agra: RakhiPrakashan, 1985.

[17] Dimitrov DM, Rumrill PD. Pre-test-post-test designs and measurement of Change. Work 2003;20:59–165.

[18] Vogt WP. Dictionary of statistics and methodology: A nontechnical guide for the social sciences, 2nd ed. Thousand Oaks, CA: Sage, 1999.

[19] Tekinarslan IC, Sucuoglu B. Effectiveness of cognitive process approached social skills training program for people with mental retardation. Int J Spec Educ 2007;22:7.

[20] Bates P, Interpersonal skills training on the communication skill acquisition in retarded children. J ApplBehav Anal 2006;13(2):237-48.

[21] Alavi S Z, SavojibAP,Amin F. The effect of social skills training on aggression of mild mentally retarded children. Proceed SocBehavSci 2013;84:1166-70. doi:10.1016/j.sbspro.2013.06.720.

[22] Pasha G, Gorjian B. The effect of training social skills on increase social development and decrease behavioral disorders in mild retarded children. Aust J Basic ApplSci 2010;4(8):4011-9.

[23] Matson JL, Taras ME, Sevin JA, Love SR, Fridley D. Teaching self-help skills to autistic and mentally retarded children. Res Dev Disabil 1990;11(4):361-78.

[24] Leblanc LA, Matson JL. A social skills training program for preschoolers with developmental delays. Generalization and social validity. BehavModif 1995; 19(2):234-46.

[25] Yakubova G, Taber-Doughty T. Effects of video modeling and verbal prompting on social skills embedded within a purchasing activity for students with autism. J Spec EducTechnol 2013;28(1):35-47.

[26] Bielecki J, Swender SL. The assessment of social functioning in individuals with mental retardation. BehavModif 2004;28(5):694-708. doi: 10.1177/0145445503259828.

[27] Salomon C. Paediatric skills for occupational therapy assistants. London: Mosby, 2000.

[28] O'Handley RD, Ford WB, Radley KC, HelbigKA,Wimberly JK. Social skills training for adolescents with Intellectual disabilities: A school-based evaluation. BehavModif 2016;40(4):541–67.

In: Intellectual Disability
Editors: Ariel Tenenbaum et al.
ISBN: 978-1-53617-866-1

Chapter 9

People with Intellectual and Developmental Disabilities: Reactions to Donald Trump Winning the 2016 United States Presidential Election

Carli Friedman*, PhD
The Council on Quality and Leadership, Towson,
Maryland, United States of America

Abstract

A common stereotype is that people with intellectual and developmental disabilities (IDD) are not capable of or interested in voting. This study examined the reactions of people with IDD to the 2016 election of Donald J Trump as President of the United States. To do so, 34 people with IDD participated in focus groups about how the results made them

* Corresponding Author: Carli Friedman, PhD, Director of Research, CQL-The Council on Quality and Leadership, Towson, MD, United States. E-mail: cfriedman@thecouncil.org.

feel and why. Findings revealed participants were concerned about the threat of harm and injustice Trump represented to themselves, their families and the country at large. Participants were also unhappy about a presidential candidate who did not necessarily align with them ideologically, especially as a threat to disability services and supports. These findings are important both for the trends they unearthed in terms of issues that impacted people with IDD, their decision making during the 2016 Presidential election, as well as to provide evidence that people with IDD are capable of actively engaging in the election process.

INTRODUCTION

According to the United Nations, “the right to vote is arguably the most important political right” (1). Through voting citizens can make decisions that both directly and indirectly impact their quality of life (2). As such, Agran et al. (2) cite voting as the ultimate act of American citizenship. Despite the numerous ways elections results can impact the lives of people with disabilities, they have historically been disenfranchised (3). Historically, in the United States, people with disabilities were denied voting rights because of a requirement of independence (3). Today, people with disabilities', particularly those with intellectual and developmental disabilities (IDD), voting access is based on state level status-based restrictions (4). The result is an inconsistent application of voting rights for people with IDD across the United States (5). However, recently there has been momentum towards increasing voting rights of people with IDD on a state-by-state basis (4, 5).

Even in states where people with IDD are allowed to vote, there are large voting disparities. Across all disability types, people with IDD have the largest voting gap compared to non-disabled people (6). Many of these disparities are related to access barriers and inaccessibility (7). For example, a United States Election Assistance Commission study found approximately half of people with IDD who voted reported polling place difficulties in the 2012 general election (6).

In addition to the physical inaccessibility of the election process, attitudinal barriers also impact the ability of people with IDD to vote.

Providers and direct support professionals have the power to serve as gatekeepers, especially as these stakeholders often do not encourage people with IDD to vote or do not see it is a priority (2, 8). This is both related to low expectations of people with IDD as well as the prominent stereotype that voting behavior of people with IDD can be easily manipulated (2). Not only does this hold people with IDD to an unfair position, because it seeks to exclude them on the basis of *others*' behavior, it also is largely untrue as research has found that people with IDD are capable of making informed voting decisions (2, 3, 9, 10). In fact, of those people with IDD surveyed in the United States Election Assistance Commission 2012 general election study, 90% of the respondents said they found voting to be easy overall (6).

Although estimates vary, up to 10 million people in the United States may have IDD (11). More research is needed about how people with IDD understand presidential elections and their decision-making processes regarding American politics. For this reason, the aim of this study was to explore election reactions from a group that is often excluded from political dialogue and research – people with IDD. Using focus groups, we examined the reaction of people with IDD to the election of Donald J Trump as president of the United States shortly after the 2016 election.

OUR STUDY

After institutional review board (IRB) approval, people with IDD were recruited (in September 2016) via electronic flyers and word of mouth through self-advocacy groups and organizations that serve people with IDD in the Chicago suburban area. Although participation was voluntary, participants were compensated for transportation and time.

Table 1. Demographics (n = 34)

Characteristic	*n*	%
Age (*n* = 32)		
18 to 24	6	17.6
25 to 34	19	55.9
35 to 44	2	5.9
45 to 54	2	5.9
55 to 64	3	8.8
Gender (*n* = 33)		
Man	22	64.7
Woman	11	32.4
Race/ethnicity (*n* = 32)		
Latinx or Hispanic	15	44.1
Black or African American	9	26.5
White	6	17.6
Asian or Pacific Islander	2	5.9
Middle Eastern	2	5.9
Native American or Indigenous	1	2.9
Other	2	5.9
Residence type (*n* = 33)		
With parents or family	21	61.8
Group home	8	23.5
Own home or apartment	3	8.8
Foster family	1	2.9
Guardianship (*n* = 33)		
Own guardian	15	44.1
Has legal guardian	18	52.9
Have trouble reading sometimes (yes) (*n* = 32)	16	47.1
Finds complicated information hard to understand (yes) (*n* = 31)	21	61.8
Voted in the 2016 election (yes)	26	76.5
First time voter (yes) (*n* = 33)	10	29.4

Note. Participants could be from more than once race/ethnicity.

Thirty-four people IDD participated in this study. Participant demographics are presented in table 1. The majority of participants were young ($n = 25$, 73.5%), people of color ($n = 29$, 85.3%), and men ($n = 22$, 64.7%). Most participants lived with their families ($n = 21$, 61.8%), compared to group homes ($n = 8$, 23.5%), their own homes ($n = 3$, 8.8%), or foster homes ($n = 1$, 2.9%). Slightly more than half of participants had legal guardians. More than three-quarters of participants ($n = 26$, 76.5%)

voted in the 2016 general election. Only a fraction of participants (n = 10, 29.4%) were first time voters in the 2016 general election. While clinical information about disability severity was not collected, as a proxy measure, participants were asked about two skills that are related to civic engagement – reading and understanding complicated information. Approximately half of participants (n = 16, 47.1%) reported having trouble reading, and slightly more than half (n = 21, 61.8%) reported finding complicated information hard to understand.

The first part of the study was a workshop run by a self-advocate held in early October 2016 about voting rights for people with IDD in order to encourage people to vote in the general election. The second part of the study, which involved the same participants, was focus groups held three days after the 2016 general election (November 11, 2016). Focus groups were selected as the method in this study because group processes can reduce the power dynamics involved in individual interviews (12); this was particularly important because of the collective history of disempowerment of people with IDD (13). Moreover, answering questions about complex phenomena can be difficult for some people with IDD (14); focus groups give participants the time to think through their answers as well as the ability to bounce ideas off each other. As long as participants are reminded to be respectful, a fruitful dialogue about a mix of conflicting viewpoints can result in group processes.

The original aim of these focus groups was to explore if, and how, the physical registration and voting process was in/accessible for people with IDD. However, following the qualitative tradition of iteration, including reflexivity and flexibility, the direction of the focus groups was "emergent and flexible, responsive to changing conditions of the study in process" and therefore driven by the participants (15). Participants were very animated about the election of Donald J Trump as president of the United States, and we used the opportunity to examine the thoughts of a group that is often excluded from political dialogue to explore why the people with IDD in this study felt the way they did.

After completing consent forms and a short survey about demographics, with support if applicable, participants were randomly divided into four focus groups. Once in their groups, the focus group leader reminded the participants that everyone is entitled to their own opinions and participants should be respectful of all opinions during the focus groups. The handful of support people in attendance were also reminded of their role to only support the participants with IDD and not participate in the research. While on occasion the support people repeated or rephrased the focus group question for the participants, they refrained from actually contributing to the discussion. In the focus groups, participants were asked their thoughts on the 2016 election including why they held the views they did.

The focus group data were analyzed using thematic analysis (16). The researcher first listened to the audio recordings of the focus groups, and then read the transcripts in order to immerse in the data. The data were then examined again line-by-line for patterns, and initial codes were generated using open-coding. The codes were grouped into themes, and revised and reviewed when necessary. The findings are presented in major and minor themes.

FINDINGS AND DISCUSSION

Themes from focus groups regarding the reactions of people with IDD to the 2016 general election fell into the following categories: threat of harm; ideological differences; dislike of personality and ways participants spoke about their feelings.

Threat of harm

According to the participants, Trump represented a threat of harm to them, both personally and ideologically. Many participants were frustrated by the ableism Donald Trump exhibited during his campaign. One participant noted, "he's making fun of the disabled." Another explained her shock that

Trump won "after all of this crap, what he said [about] disabled people…that's a bunch of BS."

Perhaps even more than ableism, the participants were particularly offended with what they understood as Donald Trump's sexism. Many participants accused Donald Trump of sexually assault. Describing him as a "womanizer" who people should not have voted for, because "he sexually assaults women." One participant went so far as to suggest Donald Trump would inevitably end up in jail specifically for sexual assault. He explained, "He's a liar…what he did. He sexually assaulted six women…he wrong. What he did, that woman, the woman that he assaulted…he going to jail."

The participants, the majority of which were people of color, were also worried about they perceived to be as Trump's racism. For example, a woman of color cautioned, "the way he [Trump] talks about people…he don't treat people right…He don't like Blacks…Ain't no [he's not] right for White [people], ain't no [he's not] right for Black [people]." Other participants connected racism with xenophobia and Donald Trump's views on immigration. For example, one participant said, "Trump hates Mexican people. They want to send the people back to Mexico. Puerto Rican people, Puerto Rican children, they want to send them back."

While participants' concerns about ableism, sexism, racism and xenophobia were certainly personal – many of the participants were directly affected by these prejudices in some way or another – they were also ideological. For example, men brought up sexism against women just as much as the women in the study; although these men are not directly affected by Trump's sexism, it conflicted with their political principles and ethical ideals.

Ideological criticisms

In addition to their stances against injustice, participants expressed a number of other ideological criticisms of Trump. Participants were concerned about the numerous ways a Donald Trump presidency would impact the issues they care about. One of the most frequently cited examples was a loss of disability services. For example, one participant declared, "I feel like something's going to happen with Trump being in office now. I feel that he might go about cutting services and that's something that we're not trying to do." Another participant countered, "I think she [Clinton] would bring more to the table than Trump would. I think she could do more as far as saving services, adding services. Doing what she can." Many participants seemed to agree similar to one participant who exclaimed, "a lot of people don't like Donald Trump because he wants to cut services."

Another topic of concern to participants was domestic and foreign policy. A handful of participants were concerned about violence, which had a particular relevance as participants were from Chicago, which has an extremely high gunshot rate (17). One participant hypothesized, "I just don't think he [Trump] would be a good president because we're all afraid that he might not do a good job with the stopping of violence." Another participant suggested, "there would've be less crime [under Clinton]." Still others thought a Donald Trump presidency would inevitably lead to war: "I feel like we might go back to war again. I feel like we have war in our own cities, so why don't we fix what's in our cities, instead of worrying about other countries?" One participant was also worried that Donald Trump would use surveillance domestically in illegal ways. The participant was particularly worried about how this might affect Black people but had trouble articulating why.

Dislike of personality

Participants also often disliked Donald J Trump because of his personality. For example, one participant acknowledged, "he wears real nice clothes and his hair be nice but it's his mouth, not his body. It's his mouth." Participants were unhappy both about what Trump says, and how he speaks about people, believing him mean. For example, a participant explained, "the way he talks about people. He is wrong…he don't treat people right." They also often expressed they believed he is a liar or a cheater. In addition to finding him unlikable (e.g., "nobody likes him"), many participants did not believe Donald Trump had the skills necessary to unify the nation, calling him "unfit." Participants also believed he was unqualified and unprepared, often contrasting him with Hillary R Clinton's thirty-years of experience in government; one participant described, "She [Clinton] actually did her homework."

Ways participants spoke about their feelings

The final theme from the study was a bit different from the first three. While the aforementioned themes focused on why participants disliked Trump both personally and ideologically, the final theme centers on how Trump's election impacted participants affectively. There was a general vitriol regarding Trump and participants felt an overwhelming sense of anger at Trump's election. Along with a number of expletives, examples of this anger from participants included violent (although sometimes sarcastic) rhetoric such a "Trump [can] burn in hell," "Donald Trump has a plane. He [should] jump out of the plane," "Donald Trump sucks. When he come to Chicago he's going to get hurt. I hate to see a man get hurt but he should stop talking about things." Throughout focus groups this anger was contrasted with an overwhelming sense of pride in, and for, Clinton. For example, one participant exclaimed, "I'm proud of her…Even though she lost the race, she's still a winner." Another participant noted, "I was on the inside a little bit crushed but on the outside I was proud about how hard she worked through the campaign and how well she was successful."

The negative affect produced by Trump's election was an expression of frustration by the character of Donald Trump and his campaign, particularly the prejudiced exhibited, and the ideology he represented. However, the way participants spoke about their feelings was also a reflection of the divisiveness of the currently political landscape in the United States. Paralleling larger conversations in the United States general population after the general election, participants expressed frustration with the Electoral College system. For example, one participant exclaimed, "the woman [Clinton] had the points. She got more votes than him [Trump]!" Participants could not understand why Clinton did not win despite winning the majority of the popular vote. Outside of the election, participants also had concerns about a dismantling of president Barack Obama's legacy. For example, one participant observed, "this whole country's going to go downhill, just like when George W Bush was our president. The country was downhill for like the last eight years. Then Obama came in. It took him eight years to turn the whole country around." Despite an overwhelming sense of frustration about the results of the 2016 general election and the bleak outlook they painted, the majority of participant planned to vote in the next election.

Limitations

When interpreting our findings, a number of limitations should be noted, particularly involving our sample. Participants volunteered to participate so there is a chance of self-selection bias. Moreover, while we hoped for a more representative sample, all of our participants supported Hillary R Clinton rather than Donald J Trump. While this may have impacted the study's findings regarding feelings about the candidates, minorities, such as people with disabilities and people of color, are more likely to vote for the Democratic party than the Republican Party (18, 19). This may be especially true in the 2016 election, which was particularly polarized between minority groups (18). It should also be noted that our participants were all from Chicago and its suburbs. Although diverse, Chicago is a solidly Democratic region. Contextual factors about Chicago may have impacted the issues that participants were most concerned about.

CONCLUSION

There is little existing research about the election experiences of people with IDD. The research that does exist mainly focuses on the access barriers people with IDD may experience when participating in voting. While attention to accessibility of the United States election process is important, it also important to understand *how* people with IDD understand and interpret elections and politics. To our knowledge, this study was the first to examine people with IDD's opinions about a presidential election. This is particularly pertinent as stereotypes often portray people with IDD as having little to contribute. In fact, proxy research using family members or support professionals rather than people with IDD is still a common method. Proxy research can be problematic because people with IDD have unique experiences and understandings to which family and professions do not necessarily have access (20).

This study recognizes people with IDD as valuable research subjects; they have "been creatively speaking up for themselves and each other" for much longer than researchers have been paying attention (13). As shown through this study's findings, people with IDD can, and do, actively engage in the political process. Participants were angry about Donald Trump being elected president of the United States. They disliked many of his personality traits, and were concerned about the threat of injustice he represented to themselves, their families, and the country at large. Participants were also unhappy about a presidential candidate who did not necessarily align with themselves ideologically, especially as a threat to disability services and supports. These trends parallel the divisiveness of the current political climate in the United States (18). Moreover, during Trump's first year of presidency, a number of participants' predictions (e.g., threats to services, dismantling of President Obama's legacy, and displays of violence, racism, and sexism, etc.) were not only well-founded but also have come true (21-24) – thereby reinforcing the legitimacy and importance of people with IDD's inclusion in political dialogue and research.

Voting is a critical form of civic engagement that allows people with IDD to contribute to decisions that will directly and indirectly impact their lives. Yet, because of stereotypes and attitudes, people with IDD's opinions and participation are often devalued (25). We believe our findings are important both for the trends they unearthed in terms of factors and issues that impacted people with IDD's decision making during the 2016 presidential election, as well as to provide evidence that people with IDD are capable of actively engaging in the election process. Low expectations about people with IDD's ability to participate in civic engagement cannot be justified. More attention to the systemic barriers that make voting inaccessible for people with IDD, and that contribute to the stereotypes that they are not interested in or capable of participating in politics is needed to address barriers and stereotypes. Doing so could directly facilitate people with IDD's empowerment.

ACKNOWLEDGMENTS

Research reported in this publication was supported by a grant from the Institute for Policy and Civic Engagement at the University of Illinois at Chicago.

REFERENCES

[1] United Nations. Thematic study by the Office of the United Nations High Commissioner for Human Rights on participation in political and public life by persons with disabilities (A/HRC/19/36). New York: United Nations General Assembly, 2011.

[2] Agran M, MacLean W, Andren KAK. "I never thought about it": Teaching people with intellectual disability to vote. Educ Train Autism Dev Disabil 2015;50(4):388-96.

[3] Beckman L. Political equality and the disenfranchisement of people with intellectual impairments. Soc Policy Soc 2007;6(1):13-23.

[4] Beckman L. The accuracy of electoral regulations: The case of the right to vote by people with cognitive impairments. Soc Policy Soc 2014;13(02):221-33.

[5] Bell DM, McKay C, Phillips KJ. Overcoming the barriers to voting experienced by people with learning disabilities. Br J Learn Disabil 2001;29(4):122-7.

[6] Schur L, Adya M, Kruse D. Disability, voter turnout, and voting difficulties in the 2012 elections. Washington, DC: US Election Assistance Commission, 2013.

[7] Government Accountability Office (GAO). More polling places had no potential impediments than in 2000, but challenges remain (GAO-09-685). Washington, DC: General Accounting Office, 2009.

[8] Friedman C, Rizzolo MC. Correlates of voting participation of people with intellectual and developmental disabilities. J Soc Work Disabil Rehabil 2017;16(3-4):347-60.

[9] Agran M, Hughes C. "You can't vote—you're mentally incompetent": Denying democracy to people with severe disabilities. Res Pract Persons Severe Disabl 2013;38(1):58-62.

[10] Schriner K, Ochs L, Shields T. Democratic dilemmas: Notes on the ADA and voting rights of people with cognitive and emotional impairments. Berkeley J Employ Labor Law 2000;21(1):437-72.

[11] Boyle CA, Boulet S, Schieve LA, Cohen RA, Blumberg SJ, Yeargin-Allsopp M, et al. Trends in the prevalence of developmental disabilities in US children, 1997–2008. Pediatrics 2011;127(6):1034-42.

[12] Diefenbach T. Are case studies more than sophisticated storytelling? Methodological problems of qualitative empirical research mainly based on semi-structured interviews. Qual Quant 2009;43(6):875-94.

[13] Owen A, Arnold K, Friedman C, Sandman L. Nominal Group Technique: An accessible and interactive method for conceptualizing the sexual self-advocacy of adults with intellectual and developmental disabilities. Qual Soc Work 2016;15(2):175-89.

[14] Finlay WML, Lyons E. Methodological issues in interviewing and using self-report questionnaires with people with mental retardation. Psychol Assessment 2001;13(3):319-35.

[15] Merriam SB. Qualitative research: A guide to design and implementation. San Francisco, CA: Jossey-Bass, 2009.

[16] Braun V, Clarke V. Using thematic analysis in psychology. Qual Res Psychol 2006;3(2):77-101.

[17] Kieltyka J, Kucybala K, Crandall M. Ecologic factors relating to firearm injuries and gun violence in Chicago. J Forensic Leg Med 2016;37:87-90.

[18] Huang J, Jacoby S, Strickland M, Lai KKR. Election 2016: Exit polls. New York Times 2016. URL: http://www.nytimes.com/interactive/2016/11/08/us/politics/election-exit-polls.html?_r=0.

[19] Igielnik R. A political profile of disabled Americans. Pew Research Center 2016. URL: http://www.pewresearch.org/fact-tank/2016/09/22/a-political-profile-of-disabled-americans/.

[20] Carlson L. The faces of intellectual disability: Philosophical reflections. Bloomington, IN: Indiana UP, 2010.

[21] Boyer D. Democratic women raise voices for Trump sex misconduct investigation after tweet about Gillibrand. The Washington Post 2017. URL: https://www.washingtontimes.com/news/2017/dec/12/white-house-rejects-criticism-trump-sexism/.

[22] Gay Stolberg S, Rosenthal BM. Man charged after White nationalist rally in Charlottesville ends in deadly violence. The New York Times 2017. URL: https://www.nytimes.com/2017/08/12/us/charlottesville-protest-white-nationalist.html.

[23] McGrane V. Trump's greatest mission: Erasing Obama's legacy. Boston Globe 2017. URL: https://www.bostonglobe.com/news/nation/2017/12/16/trump-greatest-mission-erasing-obama-legacy/OA9M4qwS2hHlOj3MGLxGxK/story.html.

[24] Next Avenue. Why big Medicare And Medicaid cuts are likely. Forbes 2017. URL: https://www.forbes.com/sites/nextavenue/2017/12/12/why-big-medicare-and-medicaid-cuts-are-likely/#40b2f01b23d8.

[25] Charlton J. Nothing about us without us: Disability oppression and empowerment. Berkeley, CA: University of California Press, 1998.

In: Intellectual Disability
Editors: Ariel Tenenbaum et al.
ISBN: 978-1-53617-866-1

Chapter 10

ABILITY OF ADULTS WITH AUTISM SPECTRUM DISORDER TO IDENTIFY EMOTIONS USING VISUAL AND MUSICAL STIMULI

Kaitlyn P Wilson**, PhD and Janet Preis
Department of Audiology, Speech-Language Pathology, and Deaf Studies, Towson University, Towson, Maryland and Speech-Language-Hearing Sciences, Loyola University Maryland, Baltimore, Maryland, United States

ABSTRACT

Social communication challenges, such as difficulty interpreting others' emotions, are central to the diagnosis of autism spectrum disorder (ASD) and are problematic across the lifespan. Neurological differences in adults with ASD have been found to underlie atypical processing of facial

---

* Corresponding Author: Kaitlyn P Wilson, PhD, Towson University, Department of Audiology, Speech-Language Pathology, and Deaf Studies, 8000 York Road, Towson, MD 21252, United States. E-mail: kwilson@towson.edu.

stimuli. Research suggests that music may assist individuals with ASD in tapping emotion. Study of the relationship between stimulus modality (visual vs. music) and emotion identification abilities in adults with ASD is in its infancy. This pilot study addressed the following questions: (a) What are the effects of group (ASD vs. non-ASD), stimulus modality (visual vs. music), and language category (expressive vs. receptive) on emotion identification performance? and (b) How do these variables interact to further explain emotion identification performance? Using a cross-sectional design, this study examined emotion identification abilities of 11 adults with ASD and 11 adults without ASD in response to visual and music stimuli. Results showed significant effects of group and stimulus modality on emotion identification, with additional interaction effects between variables. Both groups were most successful when presented with visual stimuli, and had the most difficulty identifying emotions presented musically, a task requiring concurrent processing of visual and auditory information. Adults with ASD, however, had a larger gap between their performance on visual and musical emotion identification tasks when compared to the adults without ASD. Results support the need for continued intervention for adults with ASD in the area of emotion processing, with possible treatment modalities and trajectories suggested.

INTRODUCTION

As individuals with autism spectrum disorder (ASD) enter adulthood, maladaptive behaviors (e.g., aggression, withdrawal) tend to diminish (1), yet many adults with ASD report a lack of meaningful friendships and employment (2). A key social-communication challenge of adults with ASD is difficulty recognizing and responding appropriately to the emotions of others (3), with neurological differences suggested to underlie difficulty processing facial emotion (4). The ability to recognize the emotions of others is central to successful navigation of the social world, as it dictates when and how to respond to others and plays a key role in establishing relationships in social and employment settings. This area of challenge has a clear impact on the interpersonal relationships and opportunities of adults with ASD; yet, there is limited research aimed at informing related interventions and supports for adults.

Research in neuroscience offers compelling data about underlying reasons for difficulties experienced by individuals with ASD in interpreting visual facial stimuli, showing differences in neural activation patterns between those with and without ASD during visual facial processing tasks (5). Differences in activation patterns have been highlighted for specific neural areas involved in face processing, such as the fusiform gyrus, amygdala, and superior temporal sulcus, as well as across overall neural networks (6). Additional findings suggest that individuals with ASD possess the knowledge necessary to decode others' emotions, but have impaired retrieval of this information in response to visual stimuli (7). This seems to point to the potential for alternative modalities to facilitate emotion recognition by individuals with ASD.

Research has begun to examine the potential of music as an impactful sensory experience and intervention support for individuals with ASD. Individuals with ASD have been shown to possess enhanced (compared to those without ASD) perceptual skills in response to musical stimuli (8), and may have heightened emotional response to music, similar to that of musicians, with specific dopamine receptors activated by music (9). Such findings align with music therapy research, which shows decreased psychiatric difficulties in adults with ASD following participation in music therapy programs (10).

This pilot study is a next step in examining how visual and music modalities may influence recognition and identification of emotions in adults with ASD. This study addressed the following research questions: (a) What are the effects of group (ASD vs. non-ASD), stimulus modality (visual vs. music), and language category (expressive vs. receptive) on emotion identification performance?; and (b) How do these variables interact with one another to further describe and explore emotion identification performance?

OUR STUDY

This study employed a cross-sectional design with a control group for comparison. Data were collected at one time point for each participant. Eleven adults with self-reported ASD diagnoses and eleven gender- and age-matched community control participants who self-reported no ASD diagnoses were recruited through flyers and emails distributed to participants in community-based and university programs, including a university-supported program for adults with autism. Participants met the following inclusion criteria: 18 years of age or older; hearing and vision within normal or corrected-normal limits; and ability to complete the study's consent process (approved by the university's Institutional Review Board) as their own legal guardian. Being one's own legal guardian means that, legally, one has been determined by caregivers and others to have the ability to make sound decisions about one's own personal and property related interests.

Participants self-identified their group affiliation (ASD or non-ASD) during the recruitment process. ASD symptom severity was assessed for all participants through use of the Childhood Autism Rating Scale, Second Edition, High-Functioning Version (CARS2-HF; 11), a 15-item observational scale that notes behaviors in areas such as social-emotional understanding, verbal communication, and cognitive integration. The CARS2-HF was chosen due to its recommended use with verbally fluent individuals over the age of six years (according to the test manual). The original CARS was deemed appropriate for use as a screening tool for ASD in adolescents and adults (12) and the CARS2-HF was created to more appropriately assess older individuals and those with greater verbal and cognitive abilities. The CARS2-HF was completed for each participant by a trained professional through observation of the study session and, as needed, information gleaned from others familiar with participants' behavior across settings. CARS2-HF scores were used to describe the extent of ASD symptomatology in participants, not as a means of diagnosis.

Data collection

Data collection occurred individually for each participant, with sessions lasting 20-40 minutes and taking place in a quiet room. During data collection sessions, each participant sat at a table across from a trained research assistant. Research assistants were trained to fidelity in the data collection procedure prior to data collection, with fidelity of procedures followed 100% during data collection sessions. Sessions were video-recorded for scoring of the CARS2-HF and confirmation of data as needed; however, participant responses were primarily recorded on paper during the sessions and later transferred to an electronic data file.

Following the consent process, each participant was asked to provide basic demographic information, as well as information about education, employment, and diagnoses, on a paper form created for this study. The data collection process then consisted of three phases: Picture Communication Symbol (i.e., line drawing) stimuli (PCS), photograph stimuli (photo), and music stimuli (music). The first two phases comprised the "visual" stimulus modality, while the third comprised the "music" stimulus modality. Within each phase, there was an expressive emotion identification task and a receptive emotion identification task. The expressive tasks prompted participants to verbally label the emotion they saw or heard, while the receptive tasks asked participants to point to a picture that matched a verbally-identified emotion (for PCS and photo) or musically-depicted emotion (for music). The order of the phases remained constant across participants; however, the order of individual stimuli within each phase was randomly determined a-priori for each participant through use of a random number generator. Additional information is presented below about each data collection phase.

Picture Communication Symbol (PCS) phase. For the PCS phase, a combination of black and white and color line drawings of faces was created through the use of the Mayer-Johnson Boardmaker® software program. These stimuli were chosen due to the program being commonly used in professional and research settings for children and adults with language and learning difficulties, including ASD (e.g., 13). Various skin tones were represented through the color PCS symbols. Emotions examined through use of the PCS stimuli were happy, sad, and scared. Additional emotions/expressions (i.e., surprised, angry, and tired) were included as response options in the receptive tasks. Each of the examined emotions (i.e., happy, sad, and scared) was targeted two times expressively and two times receptively. For example, participants were each shown two pictures depicting 'happy' and were asked to label the emotion for each. Next, the research assistant asked participants to pick 'happy' from the field of six PCS symbol faces two times during the receptive task. The same process was completed for all three examined emotions. A sample of PCS symbols used is seen in Figure 1 (contact authors for full stimulus set).

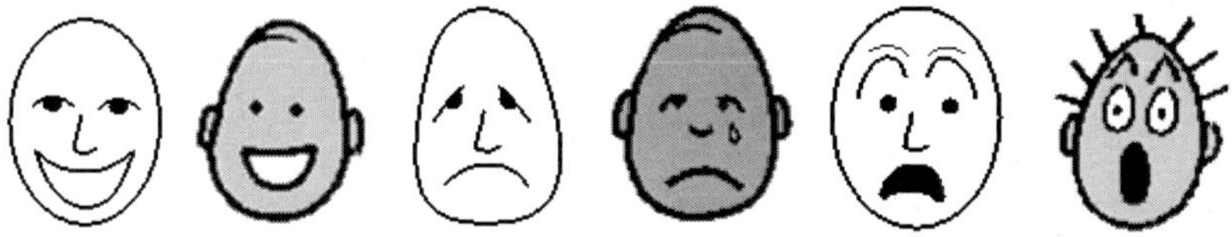

Figure 1. Sample PCS symbols for targeted emotions (happy, sad, scared).

Photograph (photo) phase. For the photo phase, Webber® Emotions Photo Cards were used. Each photograph was a color depiction of a person's upper body (starting with shoulders), face, and hair on a blue background. The photographs included people of a variety of ages, genders, and races. These stimuli were chosen because they are commonly used as a teaching tool for individuals with language and learning difficulties, including those with ASD, and because they represent a more realistic level of complexity in facial detail and emotional information. Similar to the PCS phase, emotions examined through use of the photo stimuli were happy, sad, and scared, with additional emotions/expressions (i.e., surprised, angry, and tired) included as response options in receptive tasks. Also similar to the PCS phase, each of the examined emotions (i.e., happy, sad, and scared) was targeted two times expressively and two times receptively. A sample of photo cards used is displayed in figure 2 (contact authors for full stimulus set).

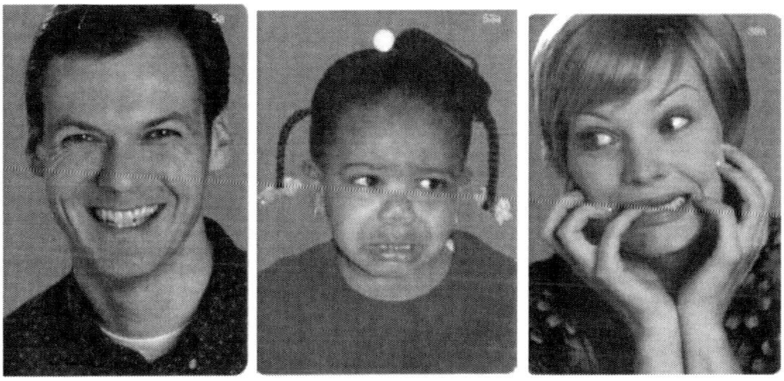

Figure 2. Sample photo symbols for targeted emotions (happy, sad, scared).

Music (music) phase. For the music phase, clips of instrumental music were used, approximating 10-15 seconds in length, with each clip previously validated for research purposes by typically developing adults to represent a specific emotion with 80% or greater accuracy (14). Clips used in this study were drawn randomly from 56 validated clips, with chosen clips depicting the target emotions of happy, sad, and scared (clips can be accessed at http://www.brams.umontreal.ca/plab/publications/article/96). Just as in the other phases, emotions examined through use of the music stimuli were happy, sad, and scared, with additional emotions/expressions (i.e., surprised, angry, and tired) included as response options in receptive tasks. Also mirroring previous phases, each of the examined emotions (i.e., happy, sad, and scared) was targeted two times expressively and two times receptively.

Response coding

In order to systematically determine accuracy of responses to expressive emotion identification tasks (i.e., wherein participants labeled emotions seen or heard using their own vocabulary) in each of the phases, Roget's Thesaurus (15) was used to identify synonyms for each target emotion. For 'scared,' synonyms listed for the root verb 'scare' were converted into adjective form (e.g., startle ? startled). See Table 1 for accepted synonyms for each target emotion. If a participant offered more than one response to an expressive item (e.g., "sad or crying"), they were prompted to choose their best response. If they reported that they were not able to pick one response, the item was counted as correct if one of the responses was correct. Additionally, responses that were merely different grammatical forms of an accepted response (e.g., sadness for sad) were counted as correct.

Table 1. Accepted synonyms for expressive emotion identification tasks

Intended emotion	Accepted synonyms
Happy	Joyous, joyful, blithe, cheerful, merry, contented, gay, blissful, satisfied
Sad	Unhappy, despondent, disconsolate, discouraged, gloomy, downcast, downhearted, depressed, dejected, melancholy
Scared	Startled, intimidated, frightened

Data analysis

Data were analyzed through a mixed factorial analysis of variance (ANOVA) procedure using SPSS 23.0 software (SPSS Inc., Chicago, IL, USA). Data were determined to meet the assumptions for this statistical procedure. The between-subjects independent variable was group (ASD vs. non-ASD) and the within-subjects independent variables were stimulus modality (visual vs. music) and language category (expressive vs. receptive). Therefore, the analysis was conducted to compare the main effects of group, stimulus modality, and language category and the interaction effects between group, stimulus modality, and language category on participants' number of accurate responses on emotion identification tasks. Bonferroni's adjustment for multiple comparisons was utilized.

FINDINGS

Demographic and CARS2-HF data were examined descriptively for participants to determine make-up of the two study groups (see Table 2).

Table 2. Demographic and CARS2-HF information for participants

	Group	
	ASD (n = 11)	Non-ASD (n = 11)
CARS2-HF raw score [mean (SD), severity group breakdown]	30.85 (6.35) Minimal-to-no ASD symptoms: 4 Mild-to-moderate ASD symptoms: 2 Severe ASD symptoms: 5	15.45 (.55) Minimal-to-no ASD symptoms: 10*
Age in years (mean, range)	28.2 (21-56)	27.5 (22-55)
Sex (count)	Male: 9 Female: 2	Male: 9 Female:2
Race (count) (note: none Hispanic)	Caucasian: 10 African-American: 1	Caucasian: 10 African-American: 1
Highest level of education (count)	High school: 8 Associate's degree: 1 Not reported: 2	High school: 5 Associate's degree: 1 Bachelor's degree: 5
Paid employment experience (count)	Yes: 6 No: 3 Not reported: 2	Yes: 10 No: 1
Diagnoses reported (count, with overlap)	ASD: 11 Speech/Language Disorder: 2 Learning Disability: 6 ADHD: 3 Mental Health Disorder: 4 Cerebral Palsy: 1	ASD: 0 Mental Health Disorder: 1

*CARS2-HF data missing for one non-ASD participant due to video malfunction.

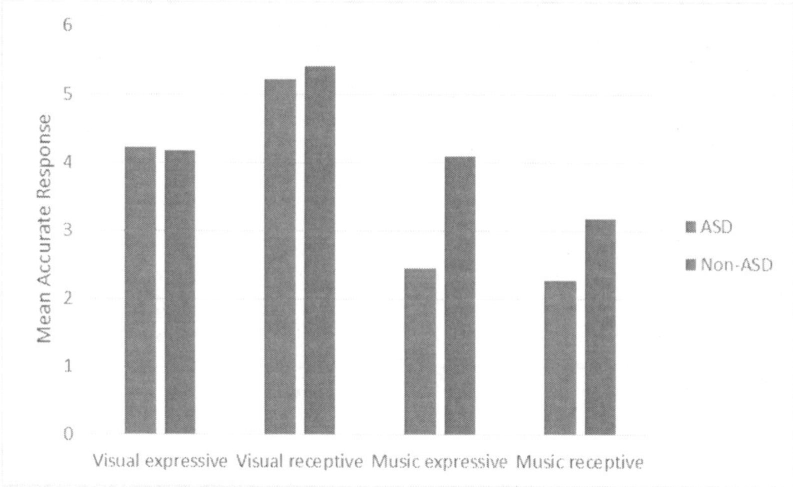

Figure 3. Mean results for stimulus modality and language category by group.

Results of the ANOVA indicated significant main effects at the .05 level for group and stimulus modality, but not for language category. Details that follow regarding means (Ms) and standard deviations (SDs) reflect scores computed on a scale of zero to six, with six being the highest possible score for each variable discussed. The main effect for group yielded an F ratio of $F1,20 = 4.403$, $p < .05$, $\eta 2p = .18$, indicating a significant difference in performance across all emotion identification tasks between the ASD group ($M = 3.54$, $SD = .84$) and the non-ASD group ($M = 4.22$, $SD = .65$), with a medium effect size. The main effect for stimulus modality yielded an F ratio of $F1,20 = 51.845$, $p < .005$, $\eta 2p = .72$, indicating a significant difference in performance on visual emotion identification tasks ($M = 4.76$, $SD = .51$) versus music emotion identification tasks ($M = 3.0$, $SD = 1.36$) across participants, with a large effect size. The main effect for language category yielded an F ratio of $F1,20 = 1.656$, $p > .05$, $\eta 2p = .08$, indicating the effect for language category was not significant when comparing participants' performance on expressive tasks ($M = 3.74$, $SD = 1.12$) versus receptive tasks ($M = 4.02$, $SD = .76$) and revealing a small effect size. The interaction effects for group*stimulus modality [$F1,20 = 6.062$, $p < .05$, $\eta 2p = .23$] and language category*stimulus modality [$F1,20 = 20.639$, $p < .005$, $\eta 2p = .51$] were also significant, with medium and large effect sizes, respectively. The interaction between language category and stimulus modality is presented visually in Figure 3 by group.

DISCUSSION

This pilot study compared emotion identification performance of adults with and without self-identified ASD on expressive and receptive tasks presented visually and musically. Groups were matched for age and gender and represented similar compositions of racial and ethnic categories. Differences between groups were noted in diagnoses reported, with the ASD group reporting many more diagnoses (in addition to ASD) than the non-ASD group, including speech/language disorders, mental health disorders, learning disabilities, attention-deficit/hyperactivity disorder (ADHD), and physical conditions such as cerebral palsy. This reflects the existing literature, which reports high rates of comorbidity of ASD and psychopathologies such as ADHD and anxiety (16), physical health issues (17), and language disorders, which often affect learning (18). Similarly, group differences in education and employment experience are representative of the literature, with adults with ASD reporting lower than average pursuit of secondary education and limited employment success (19). CARS2-HF raw score means for the groups show that there was a greater than 15 point difference between groups' mean scores, indicating much greater symptom severity in the ASD group. However, the ASD group also showed a wider range of scores (compared to the non-ASD group with all minimal-to-no symptoms of ASD), with individuals falling into all three of the CARS2-HF pre-defined severity categories (i.e., minimal-to-no symptoms of ASD, mild-to-moderate symptoms of ASD, and severe symptoms of ASD). As stated above, the CARS2-HF was not used for diagnostic purposes, but these data indicate that participants in the ASD group represented a broad span of the autism spectrum.

Results of the ANOVA indicated significant main effects for group (ASD vs. non-ASD) and stimulus modality (visual vs. music) on emotion identification performance, as well as interaction effects between group and stimulus modality, and between language category (expressive vs. receptive) and stimulus modality. Effect sizes were medium to large across these findings. These results and corresponding means indicate that the non-ASD group performed better than the ASD group on emotion identification tasks, overall, and that both groups performed better on visual emotion identification tasks than they did on music emotion identification tasks. The interaction effects show that stimulus modality is a variable that interacts with the two other variables in question: group and language category. The interaction between stimulus modality and group, when examined further, indicates that the ASD group had a greater difference (i.e., wider range between means) in their performance on the visual versus music tasks as compared to the difference in scores between stimulus modalities in the non-ASD group. Specifically, the ASD group's mean performance (out of 6) on the visual tasks was 4.73 and on the music tasks was 2.36, while the non-ASD group performed at a mean level of 4.8 on visual tasks and 3.64 on music tasks. The interaction between stimulus modality and language category brings to light an interesting performance hierarchy across groups in terms of stimulus modality-language category pairings: Visual-receptive > visual-expressive > music expressive > music receptive.

Results of this pilot study presented both expected and unexpected findings. As expected, results support existing knowledge of emotion identification difficulties in adults with ASD, as compared to those with typical development. Interestingly, across groups, the visual tasks were easier to complete than were the music tasks. While we hypothesized that the ASD group may show enhanced abilities to perceive emotions through music, findings instead suggest greater difficulty interpreting emotions from music in both groups. So, although some individuals with ASD may have enhanced processing of musical aspects (8), perhaps the requirement of emotional intelligence for the current study's tasks reduced any benefits for the ASD group. Research outside of the ASD field suggests the ability to identify emotions depicted through music may be correlated with overall emotional intelligence (20), an area that is often lacking in individuals with

ASD. In considering the non-ASD group's similar pattern of performance, the abstractness of the task (i.e., identifying an emotion that is being represented through a musical composition being orchestrated by unseen individuals) may have contributed to increased difficulty with the music tasks across groups.

The finding that the ASD group had a greater span between their performance on visual and musical emotion identification tasks than did the non-ASD group was unexpected. Given the literature showing music to be a potential area of heightened perception in those with ASD (9), and findings that individuals with ASD have impaired retrieval of emotion information in response to visual stimuli (7), pronounced difficulty with the music emotion identification tasks was not anticipated for the ASD group. Again, the abstractness of the task may have impacted performance on the music tasks across groups, with those in the ASD group perhaps experiencing greater difficulties due to comorbid language and learning difficulties, and difficulties with emotional intelligence.

Similarly surprising was the finding that the overall pattern of performance was the same across groups in terms of stimulus modality-language category pairings. The literature has long indicated that individuals with ASD show greater impairment in receptive than expressive language, beginning early in language development (21), whereas typically-developing individuals generally understand language receptively before they employ it expressively. These established patterns were expected to be seen in the current study's data as well. Instead, across groups, the receptive emotion identification tasks were easiest when presented visually, but most difficult when presented musically. That is, choosing a picture that corresponded to a stated emotion was easiest across groups, while choosing a picture that corresponded to the emotion being represented in a music clip was the most difficult across groups. The combination of music and visual stimuli may have overwhelmed participants across groups, making those tasks the most complex. However, conflicting research suggests that music may instead enhance individuals' emotional experience when simultaneously prompted through pictures (22). In the current study, adults with and without ASD had the greatest difficulty with tasks that involved the most complex combination of abstractness and sensory processing (i.e., visual AND musical), suggesting that the combination of both visual and music stimuli likely contributed to all participants' difficulty with these tasks, and even more so to the difficulty experienced by the ASD group.

Limitations

There were a number of limitations to the current pilot study, in addition to small sample size. First, participants self-identified their group status without providing official confirmation of diagnostic information. While it is likely that participants were accurate in their self-report, the addition of diagnostic confirmation will be included in future studies. Furthermore, the differing levels of ASD severity noted through the CARS2-HF had the potential to influence group data, raising questions about homogeneity of groups. Additionally, while this study did match groups on multiple variables, it did not match groups on cognitive or language level. Research has shown that IQ and emotion recognition performance are not correlated unless language is involved (e.g., interpreting emotions from spoken language stimuli (23); however, the current study was not able to test for this possibility. While the inclusion criterion requiring participants to be their own legal guardian inherently implied a level of cognition needed to make one's own decisions (e.g., consenting to participate in a research study), future studies should systematically match groups using standardized cognitive or language assessment scores to control for intellectual and language abilities.

Conclusion and Future Directions

Despite this study's limitations, findings suggest directions for clinical practice for adults with ASD and point to future research efforts in this line of inquiry. First, results add to the literature to indicate that adults with

ASD had the greatest ease in accurately matching stated emotions to pictured emotions presented through visual stimuli. We can assume that this common method for teaching emotions (i.e., through pictures and matching activities) is likely one to which the adults in the study had been exposed previously. Use of static faces (vs. dynamic faces in real life) appears to be a promising tool for teaching and discussing emotions in adults with ASD. Second, adults with ASD had more success labelling pictured emotions (i.e., faces) than they did labelling emotions depicted through music clips. Previous research suggesting music as a possible tool for understanding and teaching social understanding in individuals with ASD (24) should be considered in light of the current study's findings, as they allow for a direct comparison of performance on tasks across visual and music modalities. While existing literature shows music to be a powerful tool for reducing anxiety and supporting emotional understanding in children with ASD, the current study suggests that the complexity and abstractness of dynamic auditory stimuli (vs. more static pitches or tones) like music clips may present unique challenges for adults with ASD. Further, the results of this pilot study suggest that the combination of music and visual stimuli to target emotion identification and understanding may present difficulties for adults with ASD due to task complexity and the need for multimodal processing. Potentially, the hierarchy of performance found through the modality*language category interaction effect in the current study could suggest a process for intervention progression. For example, clinicians could first work with adults with ASD on emotion identification through visual means (receptively), moving next to the more independent step of expressive identification of emotions depicted in visual stimuli, followed by use of more abstract music stimuli, first expressively (without the addition of visual stimuli as well) and then receptively (the most complex level, combining modalities).

Next steps in this line of inquiry include larger studies with more focused examination of the performance of adults with ASD on emotion identification tasks using a variety of types of visual (e.g., static pictures versus dynamic, or videotaped faces) and music (e.g., varying length and complexity of clips) stimuli. In addition, future studies should pilot interventions using these various stimulus modalities, tailored for use with adults with ASD, and should include measures of real-world social success in order to examine interventions' potential for creating meaningful change in adults' lives. With the growing population of adults with ASD and the increasingly evident need for continued intervention in social cognition and emotional understanding across the lifespan, this line of research has the potential to inform programming for adults with ASD in a vital area.

Acknowledgments

This work was completed in part through a grant from the Towson University Academy of Scholars. We would like to thank the participants for their contribution. We would also like to acknowledge the Towson University Hussman Center for Adults with Autism for their assistance with participant recruitment efforts and facilities. Finally, we thank the research assistants and students involved in data collection.

References

[1] Shattuck PT, Seltzer MM, Greenberg JS, Orsmond GI, Bolt D, Kring S, et al. Change in autism symptoms and maladaptive behaviors in adolescents and adults with an autism spectrum disorder. J Autism Dev Disord 2007;37(9):1735-47.

[2] Eaves LC, Ho HH. Young adult outcome of autism spectrum disorders. J Autism Dev Disord 2008;38(4):739-47.

[3] Greimel E, Schulte-Rüther M, Kamp-Becker I, Remschmidt H, Herpertz-Dahlmann B, Konrad K. Impairment in face processing in autism spectrum disorder: A developmental perspective. J Neural Transm 2014;121(9):1171-81.

[4] Pierce K, Müller RA, Ambrose J, Allen G, Courchesne E. Face processing occurs outside the fusiform face area in autism: Evidence from functional MRI. Brain 2001;124(10): 2059-73.

[5] Leung RC, Pang EW, Cassel D, Brian JA, Smith ML, Taylor MJ. Early neural activation during facial affect processing in adolescents with autism spectrum disorder. NeuroImage Clin 2015;7:203-12.

[6] Nomi JS, Uddin LQ. Face processing in autism spectrum disorders: From brain regions to brain networks. Neuropsychologia 2015;71:201-16.

[7] Adolphs R, Sears L, Piven J. Abnormal processing of social information from faces in autism. J Cog Neurosci 2001;13(2):232-40.

[8] Ouimet T, Foster NE, Tryfon A, Hyde KL. Auditory-musical processing in autism spectrum disorders: A review of behavioral and brain imaging studies. Ann NY Acad Sci 2012;1252(1):325-31.

[9] Emanuele E, Boso M, Cassola F, Broglia D, Bonoldi I, Mancini L, et al. Increased dopamine DRD4 receptor mRNA expression in lymphocytes of musicians and autistic individuals: Bridging the music-autism connection. Neuro Endocrinol Lett 2010;31(1):122-5.

[10] Boso M, Emanuele E, Minazzi V, Abbamonte M, Politi P. Effect of long-term interactive music therapy on behavior profile and musical skills in young adults with severe autism. J Altern Complement Med 2007;13(7):709-12.

[11] Schopler E, Van Bourgondien ME, Wellman GJ, Love SR. Childhood autism rating scale, second edition (CARS2). Los Angeles, CA: Western Psychological Services, 2010.

[12] Mesibov GB, Schopler E, Schaffer B, Michal N. Use of the childhood autism rating scale with autistic adolescents and adults. J Am Acad Child Adolesc Psychiatry 1989;28(4):538-41.

[13] Ganz JB, Flores MM. Supporting the play of preschoolers with autism spectrum disorders: Implementation of visual scripts. Young Except Child 2009;13(2):58-70.

[14] Vieillard S, Peretz I, Gosselin N, Khalfa S, Gagnon L, Bouchard B. Happy, sad, scary and peaceful musical excerpts for research on emotions. Cogn Emot 2008;22(4):720-52.

[15] Roget's 21st Century Thesaurus, Third Edition. URL: www.Thesaurus.com.

[16] Simonoff E, Pickles A, Charman T, Chandler S, Loucas T, Baird G. Psychiatric disorders in children with autism spectrum disorders: Prevalence, comorbidity, and associated factors in a population-derived sample. J Am Acad Child Adolesc Psychiatry 2008;47(8):921-9.

[17] Seltzer MM, Shattuck P, Abbeduto L, Greenberg JS. Trajectory of development in adolescents and adults with autism. Ment Retard Dev Disabil Res Rev 2004;10(4):234-47.

[18] Rapin I, Dunn M. Update on the language disorders of individuals on the autistic spectrum. Brain Dev 2003;25(3):166-72.

[19] LeBlanc LA, Riley AR, Goldsmith TR. Autism spectrum disorders: A lifespan perspective. In: Matson JL, ed., Autism spectrum disorders: Evidence based assessment and intervention across the lifespan. San Diego, CA: Elsevier, 2008: 65-87.

[20] Resnicow JE, Salovey P, Repp BH. Is recognition of emotion in music performance an aspect of emotional intelligence? Music Percept 2004;22(1):145-58.

[21] Hudry K, Leadbitter K, Temple K, Slonims V, McConachie H, Aldred C, et al. Preschoolers with autism show greater impairment in receptive compared with expressive language abilities. Int J Lang Commun Disord 2010;45(6):681-90.
[22] Baumgartner T, Esslen M, Jäncke L. From emotion perception to emotion experience: Emotions evoked by pictures and classical music. Int J Psychophysiol 2006;60(1):34-43.
[23] Golan O, Baron-Cohen S, Hill JJ, Rutherford MD. The 'Reading the Mind in the Voice' test-revised: A study of complex emotion recognition in adults with and without autism spectrum conditions. J Autism Dev Disord 2007;37(6):1096-1106.
[24] Quintin EM, Bhatara A, Poissant H, Fombonne E, Levitin DJ. Emotion perception in music in high-functioning adolescents with autism spectrum disorders. J Autism Dev Disord 2011;41(9):1240-55.

Resources

Mayer-Johnson, 2100 Wharton Street, Suite 400, Pittsburgh, PA 15203, Phone: 1 (800) 588 4548, Fax: 1 (866) 585-6260, Email: mayer-johnson.usa@dynavoxtech.com, Website: www.mayer-johnson.com

In: Intellectual Disability
Editors: Ariel Tenenbaum et al.
ISBN: 978-1-53617-866-1

Chapter 11

PROLONGED SURVIVAL IN TRISOMY 13: IMPLICATIONS FOR COUNSELING AND CARE PLANNING

Silpa Nadella, MD, Stephanie Ling, DO, Anju Patel, MD, Meveshni Govender, MD and Dilip R. Patel*, MD

Department of Pediatric and Adolescent Medicine,
Western Michigan University Homer Stryker
MD School of Medicine, Kalamazoo, Michigan, United States

ABSTRACT

Trisomy 13 occurs in approximately 1 in 5,000-10,000 live births and fewer than 10% of infants survive till age 2 years. However, some do survive into their 20s. This has direct implications for parental counseling and medical care planning. Patients who survive beyond childhood

* Corresponding Author: Professor Dilip R Patel, MD, MBA, MPH, Chair, Department of Pediatric and Adolescent Medicine, Western Michigan University Homer Stryker MD School of Medicine, 1000 Oakland Drive, D48G, Kalamazoo, MI 49008-1284, United States. E-mail dilip.patel@med.wmich.edu.

require multidisciplinary care to address multiple medical and psychosocial issues associated with trisomy 13. We present a case of a 20 year old male who we have followed in our clinic since infancy.

INTRODUCTION

Trisomy 13, which is also known as Patau's syndrome, occurs in approximately 1 in 5,000 – 10,000 live births with fewer than 10% of infants reaching twelve months of age (1-3). In the past, the condition has been considered to be non-survivable, for which there was generally a plan towards non-intervention and palliative care. Despite this, there have been several long-term survivors documented in the literature for which the approach to these infants is being shifted from a conventional approach of comfort care and palliative care to advances in parental autonomy (4-6). Counseling of guardians should include accurate survival data of individuals affected with trisomy 13 and the decision to medically and surgically intervene or not intervene should be respected and supported with the goal for the physician and family to be in agreement on management of the infant (6).

CASE STORY

A 20-year-old African-American male with Trisomy 13 initially presented to our multidisciplinary clinic at six months of age. Our clinic team has been following him since infancy. His medical history is significant for pulmonary hypoplasia, bicuspid aorta, renal cyst, cleft lip and plate, visual and hearing deficits, and type 1 diabetes mellitus. Surgical history includes a bilateral inguinal hernia repair, abdominal exploration of undescended testes, removal of postaxial digits, and cleft palate repair. He currently functions developmentally at 8-9 years of age. Relevant physical examination findings include microcephaly, large, sloping forehead, hypertelorism, narrow palpebral fissures, low set ears, narrow philtrum, mild retrognathia, moderate throracolumbar scoliosis, micropenis, ulnar deviation of wrists, long tapering fingers and toes; surgically repaired polydactyly, hypertonicity with flexor contractures at hips, knees, and elbows. His nutritional needs are met orally with pureed foods, and patient has never required a G-tube. He is nonverbal, but can indicate his needs by gestures to his mother who is primary care giver. He also understands 1-2 word commands. Because of cognitive limitations he does not have voluntary bowel or bladder control. He receives regular physical, occupational and speech therapy. He needs to use wheelchair for mobility. He is being followed regularly in the diabetes clinic for management of his type 1 diabetes which is generally well controlled with insulin. His care is provided in a multidisciplinary team clinic setting. The disciplines in the team include neurodevelopmental pediatrics, orthopedic surgery, plastic surgery, oral surgery, medical social work, nutrition, psychology, physical therapy, occupational therapy, speech therapy, orthoptist, nursing, care coordinator and full parental participation.

DISCUSSION

Trisomy 13 was first observed by the Danish physician Thomas Bartholin (1616-1680) in 1657, but the chromosomal nature of the disease was determined by Klaus Patau (1908-1975) in 1960, when he first reported the extra chromosome 13. Klaus Patau was a German-born American geneticist, who received his PhD from the University of Berlin in 1936, worked from 1938 to 1939 in London and then returned to Germany, where he worked at the Kaiser Wilhelm Institute for Biology until 1947. He emigrated to the United States in 1948 and obtained American citizenship. Although factors contributing to genetic etiology are not known, advanced maternal age is associated with trisomy 13 (2).

A study of Baty et al. (7) used parental questionnaires and medical records from 98 families with trisomy 18 and 32 families with trisomy 13. Data from the surveys provided insight into multiple differences between pregnancies that produced trisomy 18 and trisomy 13 children when comparing them to infants in the general population. Mean parental ages have been found to be higher in trisomy 13 and 18 than in pregnancies in the general population. The average general population maternal age is 26 years, which increases to about 31 years in families with affected children. Individuals who are affected tend to have a preponderance of C-section and breech deliveries when compared to the general population, for which reasons are unknown (7, 8).

Common causes of death in children with trisomy 13 include severe brain malformation, cardiopulmonary arrest, congenital heart disease, sepsis, pneumonia and withdrawal of life support (7, 9). The factors contributing to long term survival have not been clearly elucidated as there are limited studies due to the fact that survival rates are so low (10). With the increasing number of long-term survivors with trisomy 13, it is important for counseling to begin once diagnosis is made, whether it is prenatally or postnatally. The family should be given accurate results regarding survival, and the fact that there is long-term survival associated with this condition should be discussed. Management goals and plans should be made as soon as the diagnosis is made, and accurate information regarding the infant's survival should be provided to the family at all times. A study conducted by Janvier et al. (11), in which surveys were given to the parents of over 250 children affected with trisomy 13 or trisomy 18, described the impact the healthcare system had on their child's diagnosis and how their child affected their lives. Overall 98% of parents' stated that their child, who was affected, has enriched their life regardless of how long the child survived, and 99% of parents described their child to be happy.

CONFLICT OF INTEREST

The authors of this study have no potential conflicts of interest to disclose.

REFERENCES

[1] Bruns D. Birth history, physical characteristics, and medical conditions in long-term survivors with full trisomy 13. Am J Med Genet A 2011;155A:2634-40.

[2] Jones KL. Trisomy 13 syndrome. In: Smith's recognizable patterns of human malformation, sixth ed. Philadelphia, PA: Elsevier,2006:18-9.

[3] Carey JC. Perspectives on the care and management of infants with trisomy 18 and trisomy 13: striving for balance. Curr Opin Pediatr 2012;24:672-8.

[4] Peroos S, Forsythe E, Pugh JH, Arthur-Farraj P, Hodes D. Longevity and Patau syndrome: What determines survival? BMJ Case Rep 2012;2012. pii: bcr0620114381. doi: 10.1136/bcr-06-2011-4381.

[5] Redheendran R, Neu RL, Bannerman RM. Long survival in trisomy-13-syndrome: 21 cases including prolonged survival in two patients 11 and 19 years old. Am J Med Genetics 1981;8:167-72.

[6] Merritt AT, Catlin A, Wool C, Peverini R, Goldstein M, Oshiro B. Trisomy 18 and trisomy 13. NeoReviews 2012;12:e40-8

[7] Baty BJ, Black BL, Carey JC. Natural history of trisomy 18 and trisomy 13: Growth, physical assessment, medical histories, survival, and recurrence risk. Am J Med Genetics 1994;49:175-88.

[8] Lorenz JM, Hardart GE. Evolving medical and surgical management of infants with trisomy 18. Curr Opin Pediatr 2014;26:169-76.

[9] Hsiang-Yu L. Clinical characteristics and survival of Trisomy 13 in a medical center in Taiwan, 1985-2004. Pediatr Int 2007;49.380-6.

[10] Rasmussen SA, Wong LY, Yang Q, May KM, Friedman JM. Population-based analyses of mortality in trisomy 13 and trisomy 18. Pediatrics 2003;111:777-84.

[11] Janvier A, Farlow B, Wilfond BS. The experience of families with children with trisomy 13 and 18 in social networks. Pediatrics 2012;130:293-8.

SECTION TWO: ACKNOWLEDGMENTS

In: Intellectual Disability
Editors: Ariel Tenenbaum et al.
ISBN: 978-1-53617-866-1

Chapter 12

About the Editors

Ariel Tenenbaum, MD is the director of the Center for Children with Chronic Diseases at the Hadassah-Hebrew University Medical Center at the Mount Scopus Campus, Jerusalem, Israel. He graduated the Hadassah-Hebrew University Medical School and after pediatric residency at the Department of Pediatrics at Mount Scopus Campus, he continued his work at the hospital as a senior pediatric consultant and teacher of medical students. In 2004 he was appointed the head of the new Israeli Down syndrome program in the hospital. In 2005 he started the pre-adoption clinic together with Professor Isaiah D. Wexler. In 2012 he opened the Hadassah Intellectual and Developmental Disability Multidisciplinary Evaluation Center in collaboration with the Ministry of Social Affairs. He co-founded the Disability Studies Center at the Hebrew University, where he teaches students from humanities and social studies. He was recently appointed as a child development consultant. In 2019 he was elected to the Israeli Pediatric Association Committee and serves as its scientific secretary. His main research topics are disabilities, adoption, chronic diseases and general pediatrics. He has published numerous book chapters, edited several books, and published dozens of scientific articles in international journals. E-mail: tene@hadassah.org.il

Joav Merrick, MD, MMedSci, DMSc, born and educated in Denmark is professor of pediatrics, Division of Pediatrics, Hadassah Hebrew University Medical Center, Mt Scopus Campus, Jerusalem, Israel and Kentucky Children's Hospital, University of Kentucky, Lexington, Kentucky United States and professor of public health at the Center for Healthy Development, School of Public Health, Georgia State University, Atlanta, United States, the former medical director of the Health Services, Division for Intellectual and Developmental Disabilities, Ministry of Social Affairs and Social Services, Jerusalem, the founder and director of the National Institute of Child Health and Human Development in Israel. Numerous publications in the field of pediatrics, child health and human development, rehabilitation, intellectual disability, disability, health, welfare, abuse, advocacy, quality of life and prevention. Received the Peter Sabroe Child Award for outstanding work on behalf of Danish Children in 1985 and the International LEGO-Prize ("The Children's Nobel Prize") for an extraordinary contribution towards improvement in child welfare and well-being in 1987. In 2017 appointed a Kentucky Colonel by the Commonwealth of Kentucky, the highest honor the governor can bestow to a person. E-mail: jmerrick@zahav.net.il

In: Intellectual Disability
Editors: Ariel Tenenbaum et al.
ISBN: 978-1-53617-866-1

Chapter 13

About the Center for Children with Chronic Diseases and Down Syndrome Center Jerusalem, Israel, Department of Pediatrics, Mt Scopus Campus, Hadassah Hebrew University Medical Center, Jerusalem, Israel

Chronic illnesses are common among children. These conditions last longer than a year and require continuous medical care and special needs. It is estimated that 10-20% of children in developed countries have one or more chronic condition. Advances in medicine and technology lead to an increase in the survival rate and longevity of children with chronic diseases and special needs. The severity of different chronic illnesses is variable, but there are many similarities. The child with a chronic illness faces physical, social, and emotional challenges. Therefore, medical care is not sufficient without rehabilitative service and emotional care for the child and his family.

Chronic illnesses are time and energy consuming. These children go through treatments, procedures and many healthcare visits. At home they often continue treatments as well, e.g., physiotherapy, breathing support machines and medications. This lifestyle may have detrimental effect on the child's social and emotional well-being, and similarly affect his parents and siblings.

CENTER FOR CHILDREN WITH CHRONIC DISEASES

The aim of the Center for Children with Chronic Diseases at the Hadassah-Hebrew University Medical Center at the Mount Scopus Campus, Jerusalem, is to enhance medical care, comfort and well-being of patients and their families in the hospital and beyond. The center provides integrated and comprehensive care for these patients. This includes extensive support services and helping their families cope with the burden of care.

Numerous pediatric specialty programs and medical divisions have been established in the center to care for specific chronic conditions; among them are cystic fibrosis, Down syndrome, diabetes mellitus, familial dysautonomia, neuromuscular diseases, rheumatic diseases, feeding disorders and metabolic diseases. All these programs include evaluation and support from common services in the center: Nursing, nutrition, psycho-social care, speech therapy, physiotherapy and more.

The center works as a "one stop shop" for these children; As many services as possible, under one roof, on the same visit. Centralizing the care enables parents to come to one location to receive care. The physicians and nurses coordinate the care of the children thereby alleviating some of the burden of care off the families.

Children who are included in the programs of the center usually need returning visits to various medical specialists, consultations by multidisciplinary health professionals and performing diagnostic tests e.g., blood work, x-rays and respiratory functions. Some children may need hospitalization or palliative care. The center can concentrate all diagnostic and follow-up testing, medical surveillance and treatment in the hands of an experienced staff who knows the child and his unique situation.

The center is situated close to the entrance of the hospital and the families can access it without going through the main hospital building. In the center there are ten rooms for consultations. In addition, there are dedicated rooms for tests, e.g., respiratory functions, blood tests, sweat test and more. There is a large space with eight beds for continuous treatments, for example intravenous immunoglobulins and biological medications. In this space several unique tests are performed as well, for example growth hormone test and allergy challenge tests. There is also a special room for procedures, in which children can go through painful treatments with appropriate anesthetics and surveillance.

A special classroom in the center is operated by the ministry of education. In the classroom, children can continue their studies or play and interact with other children, in arts and crafts and many other programs.

The center is surrounded by a large healing garden that is partially maintained by the children themselves.

Conclusion

In conclusion, we believe that the "all inclusive" model of a center for children with chronic conditions is beneficial for the children and their families in terms of health and quality of life, and that this model is currently the best service for them.

Contact

Ariel Tenenbaum, MD, Isaiah D Wexler, MD, PhD
Center for Children with Chronic Diseases, Department of Pediatrics, Mt Scopus Campus, Hadassah Hebrew University Medical Center, Jerusalem, Israel
E-mail: TENE@hadassah.org.il

In: Intellectual Disability
Editors: Ariel Tenenbaum et al.
ISBN: 978-1-53617-866-1

Chapter 14

ABOUT THE NATIONAL INSTITUTE OF CHILD HEALTH AND HUMAN DEVELOPMENT IN ISRAEL

The National Institute of Child Health and Human Development (NICHD) in Israel was established in 1998 as a virtual institute under the auspicies of the Medical Director, Ministry of Social Affairs and Social Services in order to function as the research arm for the Office of the Medical Director. In 1998 the National Council for Child Health and Pediatrics, Ministry of Health and in 1999 the Director General and Deputy Director General of the Ministry of Health endorsed the establishment of the NICHD.

MISSION

The mission of a National Institute for Child Health and Human Development in Israel is to provide an academic focal point for the scholarly interdisciplinary study of child life, health, public health, welfare, disability, rehabilitation, intellectual disability and related aspects of human development. This mission includes research, teaching, clinical work, information and public service activities in the field of child health and human development.

SERVICE AND ACADEMIC ACTIVITIES

Over the years many activities became focused in the south of Israel due to collaboration with various professionals at the Faculty of Health Sciences (FOHS) at the Ben Gurion University of the Negev (BGU). Since 2000 an affiliation with the Zusman Child Development Center at the Pediatric Division of Soroka University Medical Center has resulted in collaboration around the establishment of the Down Syndrome Clinic at that center. In 2002 a full course on "Disability" was established at the Recanati School for Allied Professions in the Community, FOHS, BGU and in 2005 collaboration was started with the Primary Care Unit of the faculty and disability became part of the master of public health course on "Children and society". In the academic year 2005-2006 a one semester course on "Aging with disability" was started as part of the master of science program in gerontology in our collaboration with the Center for Multidisciplinary Research in Aging. In 2010 collaborations with the Division of Pediatrics, Hadassah Hebrew University Medical Center, Jerusalem, Israel around the National Down Syndrome Center and teaching students and residents about intellectual and developmental disabilities as part of their training at this campus.

RESEARCH ACTIVITIES

The affiliated staff have over the years published work from projects and research activities in this national and international collaboration. In the year 2000 the International Journal of Adolescent Medicine and Health and in 2005 the International Journal on Disability and Human Development of De Gruyter Publishing House (Berlin and New York) were affiliated with the National Institute of Child Health and Human Development. From 2008 also the International Journal of Child Health and Human Development (Nova Science, New York), the International Journal of Child and Adolescent Health (Nova Science) and the Journal of Pain Management (Nova Science) affiliated and from 2009 the International Public Health Journal (Nova Science) and Journal of Alternative Medicine Research (Nova Science). All peer-reviewed international journals.

NATIONAL COLLABORATIONS

Nationally the NICHD works in collaboration with the Faculty of Health Sciences, Ben Gurion University of the Negev; Department of Physical Therapy, Sackler School of Medicine, Tel Aviv University; Autism Center, Assaf HaRofeh Medical Center; National Rett and PKU Centers at Chaim Sheba Medical Center, Tel HaShomer; Department of Physiotherapy, Haifa University; Department of Education, Bar Ilan University, Ramat Gan, Faculty of Social Sciences and Health Sciences; College of Judea and Samaria in Ariel and in 2011 affiliation with Center for Pediatric Chronic Diseases and National Center for Down Syndrome, Department of Pediatrics, Hadassah Hebrew University Medical Center, Mount Scopus Campus, Jerusalem.

INTERNATIONAL COLLABORATIONS

Internationally with the Department of Disability and Human Development, College of Applied Health Sciences, University of Illinois at Chicago; Strong Center for Developmental Disabilities, Golisano Children's Hospital at Strong, University of Rochester School of Medicine and Dentistry, New York; Centre on Intellectual Disabilities, University of Albany, New York; Centre for Chronic Disease Prevention and Control, Health Canada, Ottawa; Chandler Medical Center and Children's Hospital,

Kentucky Children's Hospital, Section of Adolescent Medicine, University of Kentucky, Lexington; Chronic Disease Prevention and Control Research Center, Baylor College of Medicine, Houston, Texas; Division of Neuroscience, Department of Psychiatry, Columbia University, New York; Institute for the Study of Disadvantage and Disability, Atlanta; Center for Autism and Related Disorders, Department Psychiatry, Children's Hospital Boston, Boston; Department of Pediatric and Adolescent Medicine, Western Michigan University Homer Stryker MD School of Medicine, Kalamazoo, Michigan, United States; Department of Paediatrics, Child Health and Adolescent Medicine, Children's Hospital at Westmead, Westmead, Australia; International Centre for the Study of Occupational and Mental Health, Düsseldorf, Germany; Centre for Advanced Studies in Nursing, Department of General Practice and Primary Care, University of Aberdeen, Aberdeen, United Kingdom; Quality of Life Research Center, Copenhagen, Denmark; Nordic School of Public Health, Gottenburg, Sweden, Scandinavian Institute of Quality of Working Life, Oslo, Norway; The Department of Applied Social Sciences (APSS) of The Hong Kong Polytechnic University Hong Kong.

Targets

Our focus is on research, international collaborations, clinical work, teaching and policy in health, disability and human development and to establish the NICHD as a permanent institute in Israel in order to conduct model research.

Contact

Professor Joav Merrick, MD, MMedSci, DMSc
National Institute of Child Health and Human Development,
Jerusalem, Israel.
E-mail: jmerrick@zahav.net.il

Section Three: Index

INDEX

C

D

E

F

G

O

P

Q

R

T

U

V

W

Y